Mind and Body in Health and Harmony in the Asian Systems of Medicine

Mind and Body in Health and Harmony in the Asian Systems of Medicine

edited by

RANJIT ROY CHAUDHURY

KAPILA VATSYAYAN

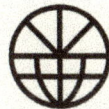

INDIA INTERNATIONAL CENTRE

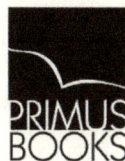

PRIMUS BOOKS

PRIMUS BOOKS

An imprint of Ratna Sagar P. Ltd.
Virat Bhavan
Mukherjee Nagar Commercial Complex
Delhi 110 009

Offices at

CHENNAI   LUCKNOW

AGRA   AHMEDABAD   BANGALORE   COIMBATORE
DEHRADUN   GUWAHATI   HYDERABAD   JAIPUR   JALANDHAR
KANPUR   KOCHI   KOLKATA   MADURAI   MUMBAI
PATNA   RANCHI   VARANASI

First published 2017

ISBN: 978-93-84092-02-3 (hardback)
ISBN: 978-93-84092-74-0 (POD)
ISBN: 978-93-84092-75-7 (e-book)

Published by Primus Books

Laser typeset by Guru Typograph Technology
Crossings Republic, Ghaziabad 201 009

In fond memory of
RANJIT ROY CHAUDHURY

Contents

Editors and Contributors

RANJIT ROY CHAUDHURY was Professor of Pharmacology, National Academy of Medical Sciences, New Delhi.

KAPILA VATSYAYAN is Chairperson, IIC-International Research Division, India International Centre, New Delhi.

C.R. AGNIVES is Editor-in-Chief, *Kerala Ayurveda Vaidyam*, the quarterly journal of the Kerala Ayurveda Academy, Aluva.

K.M.Y. AMIN is Professor of Pharmacology, Faculty of Unani Medicine, Aligarh Muslim University, Aligarh.

ESWARA DAS is Consultant Adviser (Homeopathy), Department of AYUSH, Government of India.

P.S. JOSHI is Head of Department of Medicine and Cardiology, Maharaja Sawan Singh Charitable Hospital, Beas, Amritsar.

TSULTRIM KALSANG is Senior Consultant, Tibetan Medical and Astro-Science Institute, Dharamshala.

SUDHIR K. KHANDELWAL is Professor, Department of Psychiatry, All India Institute of Medical Sciences, New Delhi.

NAMDOL LHAMO taught ar Tibetan Medical and Astro-Science Institute, Dharamshala.

B.T. CHINDANANDA MURTHY is former Director, Central Council for Yoga and Naturopathy, Bengaluru.

AUNG MYINT is former Director-General, Department of Traditional Medicine, Myanmar.

MOHAMMAD QASIM is a Specialist in Homeopathy, New Delhi.

T.I. RADHAKRISHNAN is Neuro-Physician, and former President, Indian Medical Association, Thrissur.

R.S. RAMASWAMY is Professor and Head, Department of Sirappu Maruthuvam, National Institute of Siddha, Chennai.

RAMESH P.R. is CMO and Superintendent, Arya Vaidya Sala, Kottakkal.

VIJAYALAKSHMI RAVINDRANATH is Professor and Chair, Centre for Neuro-Science, Indian Institute of Science, Bengaluru.

G.D. SUMANAPALA is Chair, Department of Pali and Buddhist Studies, University of Kelaniya.

CHARAS SUWANWELA is Professor Emeritus, Faculty of Medicine, Chulalongkorn University, Bangkok.

P.N. TANDON is President, National Brain Research Centre, Gurgaon.

Preface

SINCE 2003, IN ITS second phase, the IIC-Asia Project has adopted unconventional methods to explore different dimensions of Asian civilizations and cultures, and uncover their familiar and yet uncharted paths. In 2005, for instance, it organized the conference 'Sui-Dhaga: Crossing Boundaries through Needle and Thread', which explored the stitching together of diverse cultures of Asia through embroidery and textiles. Another composite programme was 'Culture of Indigo: Exploring the Asian Panorama', which discussed the issues of the indigo plant and its pervasiveness in Asia—the methods of extraction, the trade routes, the dyeing traditions in different regions and their artistic expressions, especially in the visual arts, and the political history of movements like the Champaran agitation. It concluded with a discussion about indigo in the market place and how synthetic indigo gave rise to the popular and global phenomenon of the denim jeans, as also attempts at revival of natural indigo in India, Indonesia, Japan and elsewhere. These resulted in various publications.

In 2012, the Asia Project held an international conference titled 'Mind and Body in Health and Harmony in the Asian Systems of Medicine'. The present volume is a result of this conference. It was felt that the present generation considers that medicine is only Allopathy and Western. The relationship between the ancient systems of Asian philosophy and medicine has thus largely remained unexplored. It was considered important to emphasize the fact that the Asian philosophic schools and the systems of medicine are not isolated and must be carefully studied, giving due respect to their interrelated nature. The conference saw the participation of various medical practitioners and researchers from different parts of Asia and also of those practicing what are called the 'alternative systems of medicine' in this country. These included specialists of Ayurveda, Siddha, Unani, Homoeopathy, Sowa Rigpa, Naturopathy, Yoga, Acupuncture based on the Chinese system, and also representatives of the traditional systems from Thailand, Myanmar, Bangladesh and Sri Lanka.

As far as speculative thought in India is concerned, I feel there has been a focused attention on the mind-body relationship. The mind-body relationship has been deeply investigated in the Vedas and the Upanishads—especially, the *Katha Upanishad*. In the conception of man (*purusa*), there is a keen awareness about the body of man as a representative of the human being and also of the universe. The micro-man and macro-man are related. Needless to mention that this would not have been possible if there was a lack of interest in man's physical body. It is the body metaphor only which is extended to investigate the nature of the universe. The mind-body relationship is most central to *Upanishadic* thought. The *Katha Upanishad* adopts the metaphor of a journey.

> *Know thou the soul (atman, self) as a riding in a chariot,*
> *The body as the chariot.*
> *Know thou the intellect (buddhi) as the chariot-driver.*
> *And the mind (manas) as the reins.*

> —KathUp. I.3.3

The *Taittriya Upanishad* explores the mind-body relationship using the simile of five sheaths of the mind and the body.

> *Annamaya kosha*, 'foodstaff' sheath (*Anna*)
> *Pranama kosha*, 'energy' sheath (*Prana/apana*)
> *Manomaya kosha*, 'mind-stuff' sheath (*Manas*)
> *Vijnanamaya kosha*, 'wisdom' sheath (*Vijnana*)
> *Anandamaya kosha*, 'bliss' sheath (*Ananda*)

> —TaitUp. II.1–5

Regarding *anna* or food, it says:

> *Verily, they obtain all food*
> *Who worship Brahama as food*
> *For truly, food is the chief of beings;*
> *Therefore it is called a panacea.*
> *From food created things are born.*
> *By food, when born, do they grow up*
> *It both is eaten and eats things.*
> *Because of that it is called food.*

> —TaitUp. II.1–2

All these instances show how mind-body relationships are essential to the philosophical and medicinal systems of India. This book is a compilation of selected essays read out at the conference and includes very significant contributions to further the debate on mind-body relationships. Each essay puts forward a very unique point. Dealing with the body and the consciousness, they stimulate one to wonder about the theoretical and practical similarities and differences in these Asian systems with the Hippocratic system. For someone interested in the textual traditions of Indian and the Asian medical systems, this volume will be thought-provoking.

Lastly, I would like to add that this conference would not have been possible but for the guidance and help, at every stage, of the internationally recognized medical specialist, Professor Ranjit Roy Chaudhury, a former member of the World Health Organization and who has contributed an introduction to the volume. Professor Chaudhury passed away recently and this volume is dedicated to his fond memory as a token of our indebtedness to him.

Chairperson   KAPILA VATSYAYAN
IIC-International Research Division
India International Centre
New Delhi

Introduction

THIS BOOK CONTAINS the presentations of world-renowned experts in different systems of Asian medicines at the international conference titled 'Mind and Body in Health and Harmony in the Asian Systems of Medicine', organized by IIC-Asia Project at the India International Centre from 11 to 13 December 2012. India, with its rich heritage and ancient knowledge, is home to many systems of medicine. We are fortunate to have medicinal systems like Ayurveda, Unani, Homoeopathy, Siddha and Sowa Rigpa. The conference also saw the participation of experts and researchers in Thai, Tibetan and Myanmar systems of traditional medicine. Besides this, experts in Yoga and Acupuncture further enriched the discussion. At a time when the country is embarking on a programme of holistic health, it was appropriate to hold this meeting. Indeed, representatives of the Government of India and the World Health Organization participated in the conference.

The theme of this conference was conceived by Dr Kapila Vatsyayan, Chairperson of the IIC-Asia Project, who provided a platform for the experts and scholars of these different systems of Asian medicine to not only look into the richness of these systems, but also focus on how the systems could come together and offer solutions to the various problems that people are facing today. We know that even experts in the Allopathic system are now turning to traditional systems like Ayurveda, for management of diseases such as cancer, coronary heart disease, diabetes, arthritis and bronchial asthma.

The unique feature of this conference was the attempt to look at the different components of the functioning of the body through the prism of various medicinal systems. While this relationship at the level of speculative thought and medicine could not be discussed in great detail, it was the underlying theme in many of the presentations. The two levels, i.e. consideration of the body qua body and the thought system of the mind, came through in different ways in the presentations by the specialists on the diverse medicine systems in Asia.

Dr P.N. Tandon's essay in this volume emphasizes that all Asian countries regard mind-body interaction and harmony as an essential element for promoting human health. He maintains that spiritual values are unique and different from religious values. Spirituality strives to strengthen the inner world, harmonizes interpersonal relationships and achieves the feeling of transcendence. The essays by Dr Aung Myint, Professor G.D. Sumanapala and Dr Charas Suwanwela talk about the traditional systems in Myanmar, Sri Lanka, and Thailand, respectively. Dr Myint recounts that the medical concept of the Myanmar system is influenced by Buddhist philosophy as well as its own traditions and customs. It has numerous medical treatises, a variety of potent and effective medicines and a diversity of therapies. Dr Sumanapala observes that Buddhism, Ayurveda and local traditions have shaped the Sri Lankan traditional system. Together with indigenous medical systems, Buddhism plays an important role even today in promoting mental health in Sri Lanka. Dr Suwanwela mentions that the Thai system is derived from both the Indian and Chinese systems. According to the Thai book *Kampir Samuthanvinchai*, there are ten main lines running over the surface of the human body which can be used to explain symptoms and provide treatments. These lines start around the umbilicus and each of them has branches which intersect at critical points. Essays by Dr Namdol Lhamo and Dr Tsultrim Kalsang bring out the special features of the traditional Tibetan system, based on its authentic medical text known as the *rGyud-bZhi* or the Four Tantras. The Tibetan system claims that the human body is physiologically made up of three principal energies, seven bodily constituents and three waste products. Their fundamental bases are the five elements, and mental consciousness has its perpetual continuum from that of its previous lives. The twenty-five aspects of the body have to be in equilibrium for a healthy mind and body.

In the valedictory address, Shri Keshav Desiraju, former Special Secretary, Ministry of Health and Family Welfare, noted that while the strengths of the traditional and modern systems should be combined, it is the practitioner who has to be good. This applies to many sectors, be it health or education. Desiraju also maintained that the system of identification and training of suitable students and their subsequent deployment in the field requires a lot of attention. At the end of the day, we have to keep the patient in mind who requires equitable, affordable and quality healthcare at an accessible distance.

This book contains a wealth of knowledge and information which not only brings alive our heritage of these ancient systems of medicine but also shows the way these systems can be used today for improving the physical and mental health of our population

Professor of Pharmacology   RANJIT ROY CHAUDHURY
National Academy of
Medical Sciences
New Delhi

The Human Body
Multiple Dimensions

P.S. JOSHI

WHENEVER WE DISCUSS life sciences and healing, it is customary to invoke an image of Lord Dhanvantari. Gods, repeatedly defeated and killed by their more powerful cousins, the asuras, had approached Lord Vishnu, seeking the boon of rejuvenation and the gift of immortality. He directed them to churn the primeval ocean in which were hidden the secrets of life and death.

With the Naga Vasuki as the rope and Mount Mandara as the churning rod, they churned the ocean till it yielded several valuable things such as

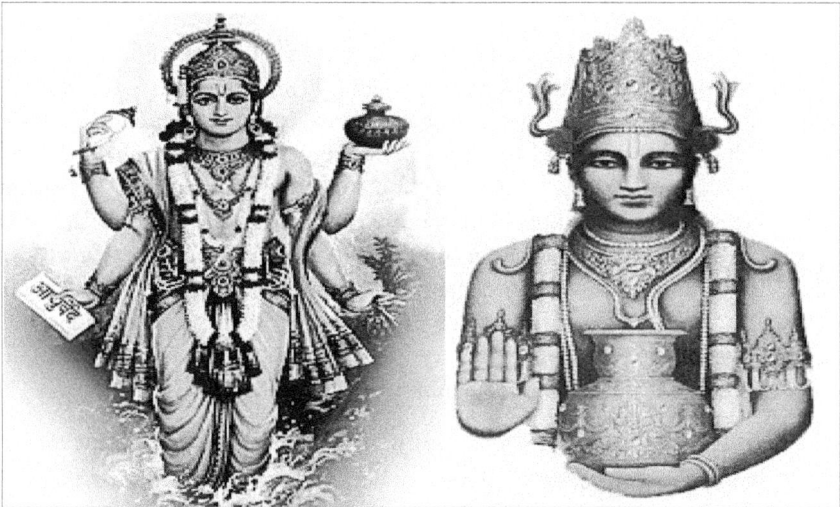

Fig. 1.1: Lord Dhanvantari and the pot of Amrit.

Source: http://www.govindrakshak.com/dhanvantari.png http://www.ayurvedic-reisen.com/images/dhanvantari.gif.

a wish fulfilling cow (*Surabhi*), Goddess of intoxication (*Varuni*), Parijat celestial tree, celestial nymphs (*Apsaras*), the moon, poison (*Halahal*) and Lakshmi, the Goddess of prosperity. Finally emerged Lord Dhanvantari, the divine physician, holding the pitcher of *amrit* (the elixir of life) which is capable of taking away diseases and death, thereby granting immortality.[1] The search for this pot and its contents has dominated my life.

Precious Human Body

We are taught by saints and yogis that to be born as a human is great good fortune as the human body is the entry to *karma bhoomi*. And only in a human birth do we get the capacity to create fresh *karmas*. All the other species—8.4 million of them—are living out their past *karmas* as *bhog yoonis*.

It is only in the human form that the Soul can realize God and retrace its footsteps homeward. None other of the 8,400,000 species has this privilege. Man alone is so blessed. Even gods and angels pine for this opportunity. The human body is the exit through which one can escape the vast prison of the unending cycle of death and rebirth thereby putting an end to all pain and misery. But alas! We forget this supreme objective and get entangled in the pursuit of the pleasures of the senses.[2]

The *Shambhala Dictionary of Buddhism and Zen* mentions the various forms of existence:

Between the various forms of existence there is no essential difference, only a *karmic* difference of degree. In none of them is life without limits. However, it is only as a human that one can attain enlightenment. For this reason Buddhism esteems the human mode of existence more highly than that of the gods and speaks in this context of the 'precious human body'. Incarnation as a human being is regarded as a rare opportunity in the cycle of *samsara* to escape the cycle and it is a challenge and obligation of humans to perceive this opportunity and strive toward liberation (enlightenment). . . . Although the gods are allotted a very long, happy life as a reward for previous good deeds, it is precisely this happiness that constitutes the primary hindrance on their path to liberation, since because of it they cannot recognize the truth of suffering.

Before we enter the human body, many of us are very clear about our purpose, which is, to evolve to a better stage of consciousness and to ultimately realize the 'Self'. However, once inside the mortal frame, we tend to forget the subject and become entangled in the day to day distractions of survival, pleasure and power. If we are fortunate enough to listen to the teachings of a master and engage in appropriate practices, there is a possibility of evolving to a higher level of consciousness so that we can become masters of our destiny.

Before we proceed, it is prudent to define some of the terms used in this submission:

Spirit: It is used to denote the supreme reality, the One, God, the source of all.

Soul: The spark of the spirit as an individual entity, *Atman*, bereft of Ego, all coverings.

Jivatman: Individual soul covered by various sheaths of creation/illusion, mind and body.

If we spend our entire life protecting our self, accumulating wealth, power and instruments of pleasure, then, at the end of our days, we are plunged inexorably into the cycle of reincarnation based upon our *karmas*.[3] 'The true value of the human body is realized after death, when man regrets that he has squandered his most precious possession. The result is that he has to go to hell or to lower births. Similarly, the Bible says that we are selling our birthright for a mess of pottage.'[4]

Peace and Happiness

Human beings have physical, emotional, mental and spiritual aspects with which they search for peace and happiness. Our physical, mental and emotional selves are only capable of connecting with the things of this material world which change and die. Because they are impermanent, the happiness they provide is impermanent. Only by developing our spiritual nature can we find a source of peace and happiness that is permanent. People refer to this fountainhead of permanent joy and peace by many names, such as God, Universal Consciousness, Tao, Shabd, Word, and so on. One way to make conscious contact with this infinite source of peace and happiness is taught by the masters who teach Surat Shabd Yoga, the method of uniting our spiritual self with the inner sound current. Their teachings are known as *Sant Mat*, an Indian phrase meaning the teachings of the saints. These masters teach a practical way of developing our spiritual nature so that we can achieve lasting peace and happiness.[5]

Spirit is Life and Deeper: Levels of the Consciousness

At the centre of life is spirit—one and indivisible. Spirit is perfection, imperturbable, the origin of all. From the one emerges all diversity, all forms from the most subtle to the most gross, all activity and complexity, the entire creation. Spirit is love. Spirit is energy. Spirit is life. Mind, matter and senses have no life of their own—they are the means by which the spirit expresses and manages itself in material dimensions. Spirit comes from a source beyond mind and matter, beyond the law of cause and effect. Soul, a drop of spirit that allows a being to be defined apart from the ocean of spirit, is the energy or power that sustains individualized life. When soul, the life force, leaves a body or living being, that body dies, disintegrates, and reverts to its original matter, dust to dust. If spirit leaves the creation, the creation disintegrates and reverts to an earlier, less-formed reality. The mystic journey of enlightenment, then, is the expansion and deepening of consciousness from life's most transient material manifestations to the permanence of its spirit-filled heart.[6]

DYING WHILE LIVING

Most of us stay in perpetual motion all our lives. Afraid of death, we fill up our time, and minds, with the comfort of busyness, with responsibilities and pleasures. We fear death because it lies on the other side of the barrier between the known and the unknown. Although it is the one inevitable event that we are all moving towards, we avoid thinking about it and desperately run the other way. We plunge into all kinds of enjoyments. We pursue money, power, and status. We submerge ourselves in our family responsibilities and attachments. But still we have the nagging realization that something awaits us at the end of it all, and that is death. Is there any way to know what is on the other side? Has anyone ever been there and come back to tell all? It would seem not; it would seem that we are all in the same situation. Yet somewhere amid the din and distractions of life is the voice of the mystics, those enlightened souls who have appeared in all religions, at all times in history and at all places in the world. These mystics teach us that if we can still our minds and take our attention within, we can transcend the limitations of the body and mind and experience God. Their process of meditation takes us beyond the barrier of death, and that is why it is sometimes called 'dying while living'.[7]

At the time of death, our consciousness vacates the physical body like a dweller vacating a building, and moves into subtle realms before continuing its endless journey of reincarnation. However, if we learn to experience this process of dying (consciously withdrawing our consciousness out of the body), we can not only learn the mysteries of death but can come back to the physical body or leave it at will. This is the way to liberation from *sansara*—the endless cycle of reincarnation to reach self-realization and God realization.

The saints or masters call this practice 'dying while living', for by withdrawing our consciousness to the Third Eye and listening to the music of the sound current or audible life stream, the mind and the soul come out of the tomb of the body and become free from it. Their attachment to the world thus broken, they forget the troubles and miseries of the world and enjoy eternal bliss.

> *Death, for the world, is the greatest fear,*
> *But fills my heart with bliss.*
>
> —*Santan di Bani,* Bani Sant Kabir Ki, p. 1365

> *Die while living;*
> *Such is the yoga at which one should labor.*
>
> —*Santan di Bani,* Guru Nanak, p. 730

Similarly, St. Paul says in the Bible, 'I die daily' (I Corinthians 15:31). The Muslim scriptures also bring out the same point, saying, 'Die before thy death'. Dadu, a celebrated saint, writes in his *Bani* or teachings:

> *Die, O Dadu, before*
> *The messengers of death arrive;*
> *What uncommon is there in dying*
> *As others do?*
>
> —*Dadu Dayal ki Bani,* Dadu, 1:191, *Divine Light, The Path,*
> Maharaja Charan Singh, pp. 60–1

Human Lifespan

In the present *yuga,* we see few people reaching the theoretical age limit of a hundred years. Out of these hundred years, the initial twenty years are lost in childhood and in acquiring basic education/skills which can sustain us financially. One-third of the entire life is lost in sleep (there are ways of using sleep and dreams for evolution of consciousness but most of us choose not to explore this option). The last thirty years of life, beyond seventy years of age, are most often not very fruitful for any energetic endeavour, as our faculties get damaged by various diseases or degeneration. So, we can see that the actual productive lifespan at our disposal may be only twenty to forty years.

This lifespan of twenty to forty years is very brief, compared to the age of numerous other entities. We are told that even gods, angels, *gandharvas,*

apsaras, maruts, vasus, Manu, *rishis, munis,* etc., are envious of us and
wish for this mortal frame (Is Dehi Ko Simrain Dev).[8] This is because we
have the human form but they have to wait for long periods before they
can hope to enter the human incarnation. It is only in the human form
that they can perform meritorious deeds and meditation which will make
them evolve to a higher level of consciousness. The average lifespan of a
god like Indra is estimated at 3.06 million human years. Brahma's one
day and night is 8.64 billion years long and the lifespan of Brahma is
estimated to be 311.04 trillion years![9] If these gods are said to be waiting
for a chance to get into the human form, then human birth must be a
very precious opportunity.

NUMBER OF SPECIES

The *Padma Purana* discusses a number of different types of life forms in
the universe. According to the *Padma Purana*, there are 84,00,000 life
form species, 9,00,000 of which are aquatic ones; 20,00,000 are trees and
plants; 11,00,000 are small living species, insects and reptiles; 10,00,000
are birds; 30,00,000 are beasts and 4,00,000 are humanoid species. Out
of all theses, only the human form is said to be suitable for self- and god-
realization.[10]

Uses of the Body

The human body can be used for multiple objectives: Enjoying different
kinds of pleasures. The human mind is always looking for pleasure in one
form or the other. Fulfilling responsibilities like taking care of parents
and offspring, and settling *karmic* debts either through finances, service
or disease are also the uses of the body. But the noblest use of the body
would be to listen to the teachings of a saint/guru/spiritual guide and use
this rare opportunity for self-realization.

The human body has multiple dimensions.[11] Most of us are aware
of only the gross physical form of our bodies. This is because of our
restricted vision and perceptions. We all know that when white light is
passed through a prism, the multiple bands of coloured light (which are its
constituents) can be appreciated. Similarly, a different form of vision has to
be cultivated to be able to see that our body actually exists simultaneously
on multiple plains of existence. A set of Russian wooden dolls, where a
tiny coloured bead is encased in doll casings of progressively increasing
sizes, can be used as a rough illustration.

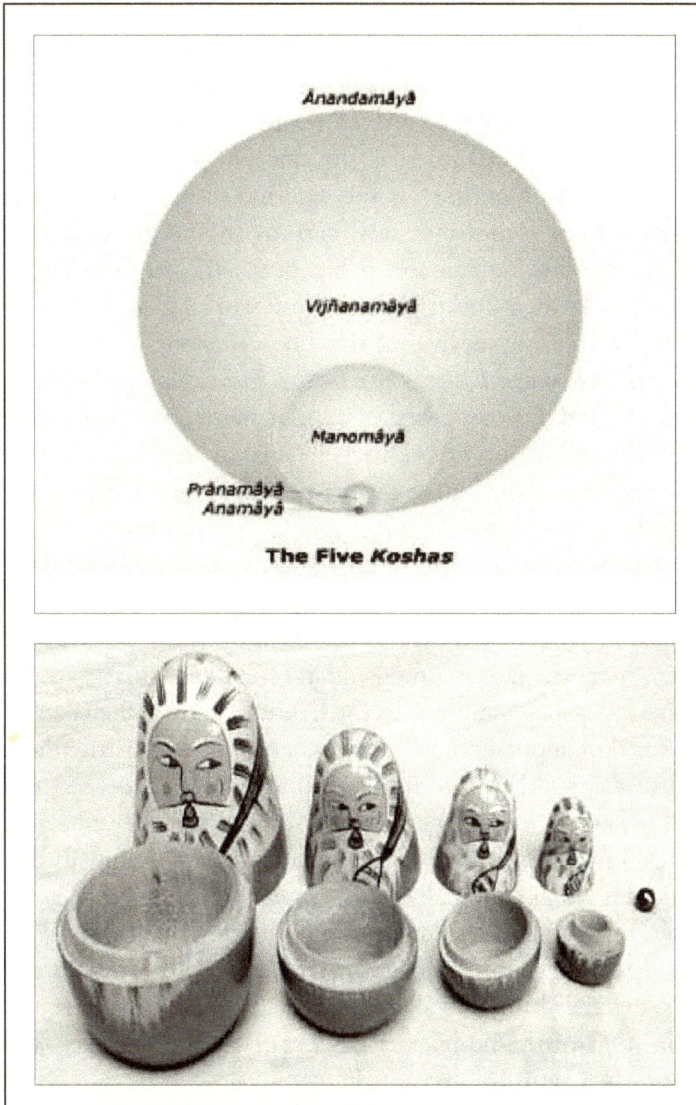

Ānandamāyā

Vijñānamāyā

Manomāyā

Prānamāyā
Anamāyā

The Five Koshas

Fig. 1.2: The Five *Koshas*.

Source: http://www.srivyuha.org/Sri Vyuha/images/koshas.jpg. The Russian dolls,
http://www.swamiji.com/images/dolls.jpg.

Rishis who meditated hard to develop the capacity to see (the 'Seers') have indicated that there are at least five major dimensions of the human body.[12] *Atman* is distinct from the five *Koshas* or sheaths. These are called *koshas* or sheaths because they cover individual sparks of consciousness (our souls) with layers of matter that the Soul needs to interact with these realms, when we enter the creation. From gross to subtle, the five sheaths are: *Annamaya kosha* (food sheath), *Pranamaya kosha* (vital sheath), *Manomaya kosha* (mental sheath), *Vijnanamaya kosha* (intellect sheath) and *Anandamaya kosha* (blissful sheath). *Maya* means composed of and sustained by and *kosha* means sheath.[13]

The gross or physical body is the one we are most familiar with. In Yoga, this is also identified as the external instrument, because with its help we move around and take actions in the physical world. As this body is the one we can see, it has been studied extensively and a fair amount is known about its anatomy, working and disease states. As food is essential for survival of this body (barring exceptions), it has been named *annamaya kosha*. *Pranamaya kosha*, also called the energy body or astral body, is composed of subtler material as compared to the physical body, and is thus not easily perceived by our eyes. However, it is tremendously important for the proper functioning of the physical body. Energy body is composed of many channels conducting energy (*prana*) to its various parts and *chakras* or energy centres, which modulate/down regulate higher energy frequencies according to the needs of various functional systems. Blocked *chakras* fail to transmute required amounts of energies at proper frequencies/intensities for functional systems they govern and disease states may manifest. In the hands of an experienced yogi, who can access and manipulate the *Pranamaya kosha*, these obstructions can be removed by very subtle means like a needle, mantra or focused attention, thereby normalizing the flow of *prana* and resolving the imbalance.

I believe the discipline of Acupuncture works optimally in the hands of practitioners who can actually see the *pranamaya kosha* with its channels and energy centres and are adepts at manipulating the flow of *prana*. The energy body can detach itself from the physical body temporarily (while staying connected through a silver cord) and one can perceive the astral dimension. Out-of-the-body experiences and near-death experiences are based upon such transitory escapement.[14]

At the time of physical death, the *pranamaya kosha*, encasing other subtler bodies and consciousness, separates from the physical body permanently, thereby manifesting the phenomenon of death. This process is usually quite painful and most people fail to remain aware during the process of death.

The process of physical death, if gone through while maintaining consciousness and awareness, can result in tremendous learning and thus provide an opportunity for controlling future incarnations or attaining the state of enlightenment. Many spiritual disciplines including Christianity, Tibetan Buddhism, Radha Soami Santmat and certain yogic traditions emphasize the study and duplication of the process of death while living, as a means to liberation.

Manomaya Kosha, Vijnanamaya Kosha and Anandmaya Kosha

Because of our limited understanding, we often equate the mind and the brain. But the yogic experience (which is based on observing the functioning and communication between the mind and the brain from a perspective higher than that of the mind), posits that the brain is used by the mind as an organ of expression on the physical plane. The brain is not the seat or container of the mind. It is the mind which is vast and contains the brain, along with the rest of the creation. This is difficult for us to comprehend from our level of consciousness even if we create a concept for it because a concept is more like a map, it is never the real thing.[15] Concepts formed from incomplete knowing and held on to rigidly, can seriously hinder spiritual progress.

In yogic terms, the mind itself is called *antashkarn,* i.e. the internal instrument. It has no intelligence or consciousness by itself. That property is imparted to it by the visiting soul/self. However, it must be appreciated that the mind is a very powerful instrument, is extremely vast and affords the consciousness an opportunity to experience creation at multiple levels.[16]

The one component of the mind is the *manaspatal,* which is like a display screen. *Manas* or the lower mind which is in touch with sensory organs, i.e. the eyes, ears, nose, skin and tongue, adds instinctual biases—likes and dislikes, pleasant and unpleasant—and projects them on the *manaspatal.* Simultaneously, all impressions, with the attached biases and emotional content, are sent to *chitta,* which is like a huge hard disc storage device and a repository of deeper levels of intelligence and consciousness as well as *Aham* and *Buddhi.*[17]

The impressions created by *manas* are analysed by *aham* or *ahankar* to determine whether the situation threatens the survival of the physical unit and also to determine if it will give pleasure or add to the power of the individual unit. *Buddhi* is supposed to discriminate and determine an intelligent approach to the data provided by both *manas* and *ahankar,* and to decide the final course of action. If *buddhi* gets influenced by both *manas* and *ahankar,* actions become dominated by instinct and ego, not discrimination. As we evolve, *vivek buddhi* manifests become capable of overriding instinctive emotional inputs and more competent at taking

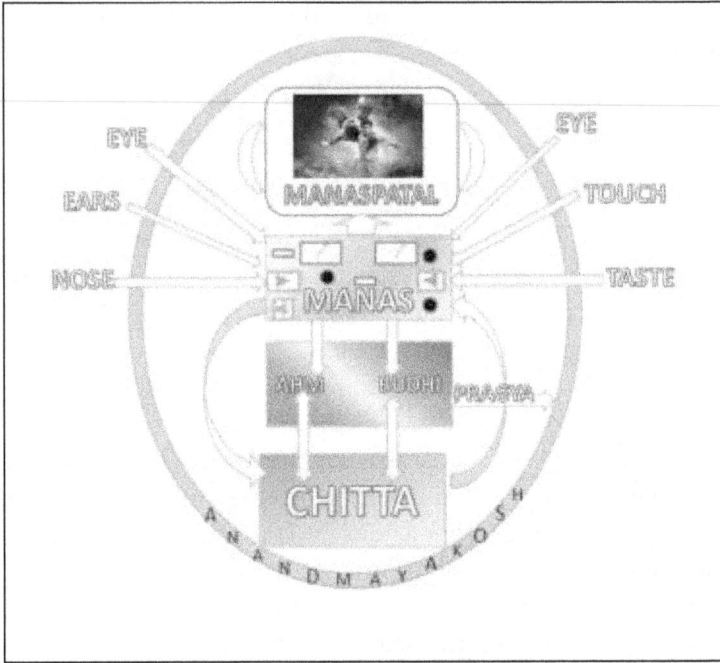

Fig. 1.3: Anatomy of the Mind.
Source: Author.

balanced intelligent decisions which are in the long-term interest of the body-mind-soul unit. When *buddhi* gets directed towards the self and takes guidance from its light in conducting the functions of the mind-body unit, it is called *pragya*.

When external inputs are cut off (closing the eyes and ears and sitting still in a quiet, darkened place), previously stored impressions from the *chitta* are projected by the *manas* on to the *manaspatal*—like a VCR in replay mode when TV channels are switched off. *Manas* with *manaspatal* and *ahankar* can be considered the lower mind/ *Buddhi*. *Buddhi* is in the domain of *vijnanamaya kosha*. *Anandamaya kosha*, emanating from the causal body, closest to the self, resplendent in the light of the self, is full of bliss.

The Supreme Source, Self and Creation

Each individual soul is a spark of consciousness separated from the supreme source. It is essentially the same as the source, but limited. When it descends into creation, it gets encased in coverings or sheaths, by the coverings of matter.[18]

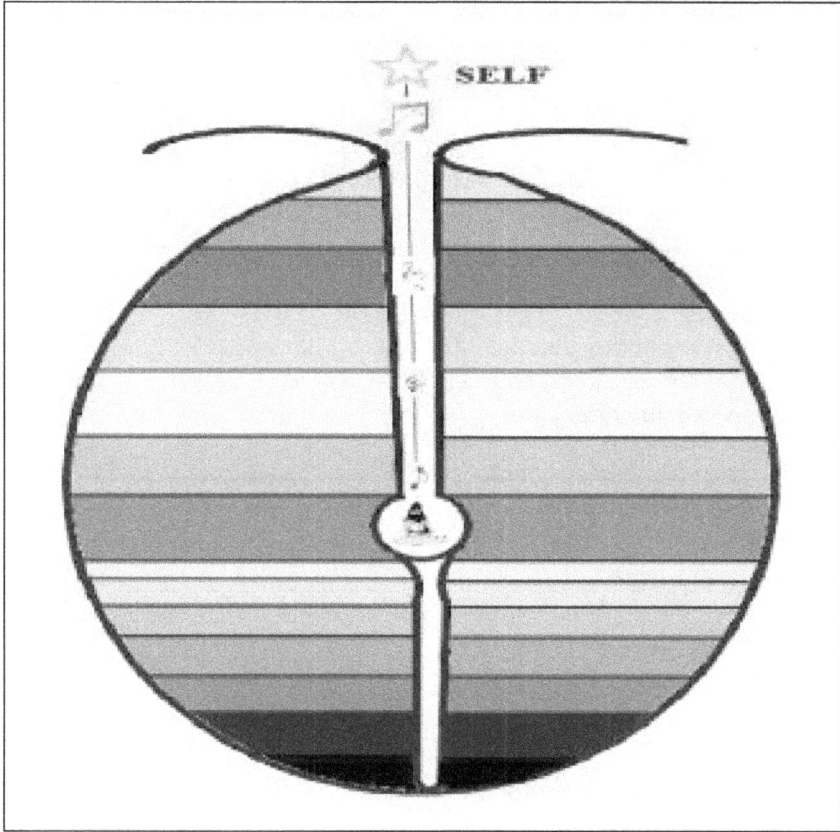

Fig. 1.4: The Source (Spirit), the individual soul and covering sheaths with plains of creation.

Source: Author.

As soul enters the creation, to experience its various levels, it acquires sheaths of different densities of matter, appropriate for each plane of manifestation. Every step in shedding these sheaths enhances our vision and comprehension with a commensurate increase in our powers. The consciousness situated at a particular level can easily see that plane, but does not have ready access to planes higher than its present station. After shedding all the sheaths of matter and mind, we come face to face with our true Self. At this stage, true *vairagya* is experienced, because although the Self is full of bliss, now its only desire is to merge with the Supreme source (Spirit) for the experience of oneness and ultimate fulfilment.

The Upanishads say: 'Know thyself'. Christ exhorted us to do the same. The Persian saints also preached this, and so did Socrates. Guru Nanak has emphasized this very truth, saying that so long as we do not know ourselves we cannot be free from the deception of *Maya* (Illusion). The saints gained this realization and taught people to turn their attention towards this goal. So long as our attention is fixed on the world and worldly objects, we are subject to pleasure and pain. But when the attention is directed towards the Lord, we cross the barriers of pleasure and pain. Then God-like qualities, which had remained latent within us, become manifest. A part bears witness to the existence of the whole. So the soul, which is a part of the Lord, merges in him as soon as it turns its attention towards the Whole. Soul is neither mind nor intellect. Mind and intellect are its instruments for functioning in this world. This is where some philosophers make a mistake. Real knowledge is the merging of the soul in the Lord, and real devotion implies the efforts made in that direction. The object of internal practice is to free the soul from its bondage to the body and to the objects of the world. This practice may be divided into three parts:

1. That which relates to the tongue of the soul and is called *simran*, repetition or remembrance.
2. That which is to be done with the eye of the soul and is known as *dhyan* or contemplation.
3. That which is done with the ear of the soul and is called *bhajan* or listening to the Shabd, or voice of God.[19]

The Role of the Guru and Meditation

Like a frog in a small pond, when we are in the physical domain, we are quite often very happy with whatever is going around us and this enjoyment of creation remains our only concern, as we are not aware of any other possible realm of existence. We have great faith in our intelligence, however limited it be. We are unaware of the inherent impermanence of all creation we see. We also do not realize that all our pleasures lead to pain and suffering, and we are caught in this prison of reincarnation without respite. We fail to recognize that we should be using this unique opportunity of human birth for realizing the Self, so that we can permanently escape the cycle of *sansara* and abide eternally in bliss.

Like the famous story of the princess kissing the frog and transforming it into a prince—the kiss of awareness is very necessary for us to truly appreciate our position in this creation and to understand the objective for which we have incarnated. Such awareness comes through the teachings, grace and guidance of the guru.

Once the frog becomes a prince by the grace of the guru, he is not to spend his time in the pursuit of worldly pleasures. His job is to strive single-mindedly to achieve spiritual evolution. A prince is the son of the king and is a king in the making—but the transformation from a prince to an effective king requires tremendous focus and effort. The recipe for that is meditation under the guidance of a guru who has already completed the journey and is familiar with the path and possible obstacles.

God-realization is not possible without a perfect Master: The Vedas, Shruties, Smrities, other holy scriptures and the Saints and Sages of all religions stress the need for a Mystic Adept for transport into subtle realms. Actually, man needs a teacher at every step from the time of his birth. He has learnt nothing without one. His first guru is his mother who teaches him how to sit, stand, walk, eat, drink and dress. Later his father, brothers and sisters take on the onerous role and he begins to prattle. When he grows a little older, his friends and playmates become his guru. Next he goes to schools and colleges where there are any number of them to teach him. Yet when it comes to learning the science of the soul—the most intricate of sciences, rarely do we search for a guru, and without one it is impossible to proceed even an inch on this path. Maulana Rum says:

> Even in the streets through which,
> You have passed a number of times,
> You often miss the way,
> If you do not have a guide.
> Beware of the way,
> Which you have never traversed.
> Never go there alone,
> Always take a guide.

Not only is it impossible to know God without the help of a Mystic Adept, but without his protecting hand over one, it may be hazardous to make an attempt at going into subtle regions. In this path, many are the temptations to lead us astray, many the pitfalls to drag us down. Without a guide, we are sure to lose the way and fall into the quagmire of delusion and danger. The Perfect Master will show us how and where to enter the body, 'the temple of living God'.[20]

Meditation

Meditation involves disengaging our attention from the objects of this creation, controlling the wanderings of the mind (which is driven by desires for pleasure materials and power) and going inside. We have to confront certain portions of our psyche which we do not accept as parts of our false self or Ego, an artificially created entity for interacting on this mortal plane of existence. Meditation needs be conducted under a realized guide. Unless we integrate the good and bad parts of our personality into one unit, accept the reality as it is and assimilate these lessons, we cannot proceed to higher levels of consciousness. The mythological story of Samundra Manthan and the holding of Halahal by Neelkanth Shiva allegorically points to such a process.

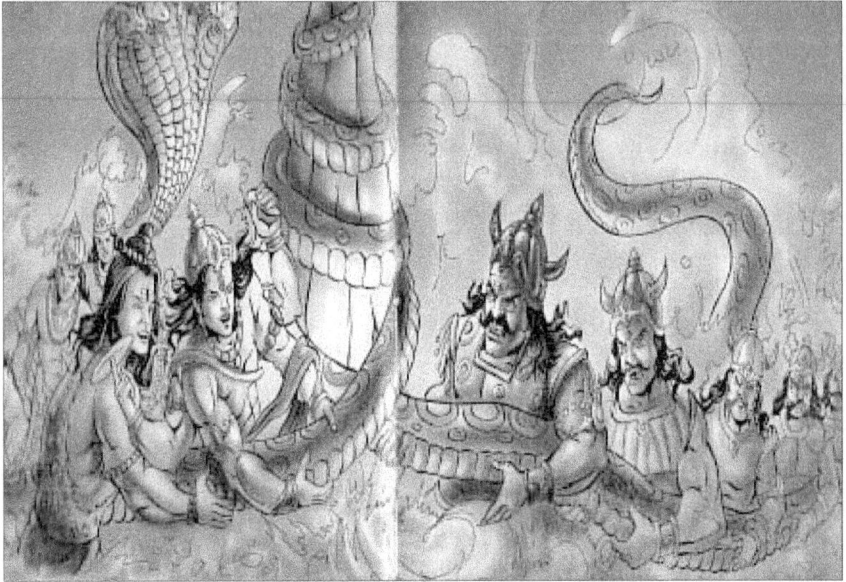

Fig. 1.5: Samundra Manthan.

Source: http://www.kidsgen.com/fables_and_fairytales/indian_mythology_stories/samudra_manthan.htm.

The process of Samundra Manthan carries spiritual connotations for me. In an indirect way, it points to one of the processes of meditation and spiritual progress. The Naga Vasuki possibly denotes Kundalini—the *manthan* of our mind is meditation. We start in a state of duality where we have the *Satvic* (devas) and *Tamsic* (asuras) as well as the *rajogun* reflected in the struggle of churning. The mind (Lord Vishnu as a turtle) forms a firm ground when the outgoing tendencies (the legs of the tortoise) are withdrawn. The mount Meru is the spinal column. After intense effort, initially poison comes out of our subconscious mind (Halahal) which is our ugly part, injurious to the ego and pushed deep into the subconscious.

This poison is held in the throat (anything held in the throat cannot escape our constant awareness) as swallowing it is injurious for emerging self-awareness (Shiva). Why hold the poison in the throat? When we hold our own shortcomings and flaws constantly in our awareness, we do not feel impelled to judge and criticize others with similar flaws. A sense of kinship grows in us as we perceive that we humans are all the same and compassion follows for ourselves and others. Once this poison is integrated and neutralized, treasures start appearing from deep within ourself. However, these are also mere distractions (as they represent *siddhis*) and are not the objective of our quest.

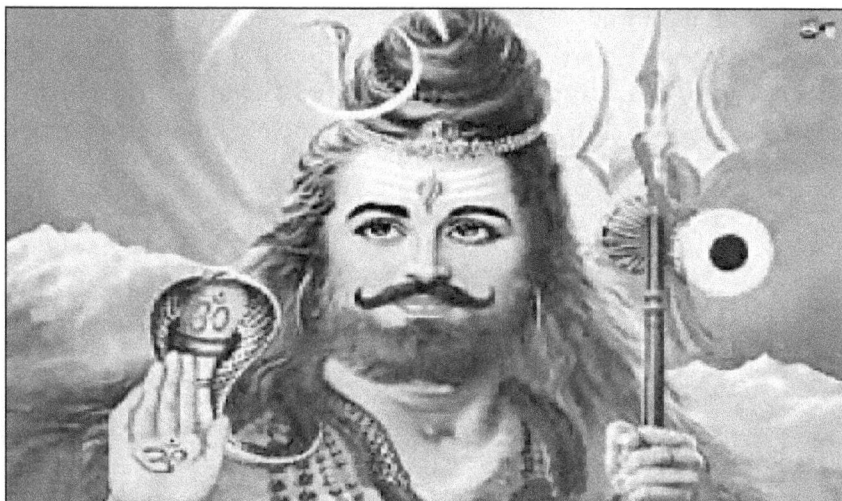

Fig. 1.6: Lord Shiva.
Source: http://www.widehdwallpapers.in/lord-shiva/jai-bholenath-hd-wallpaper.html.

Finally emerges Lord Dhanvantari—the bearer of the *amrit*—which can bestow life immortal beyond the confines of this physical mortal frame! Once this poison is integrated and neutralized, treasures start appearing from the deep. However, these are also mere distractions (as they represent *siddhis*) and are not the objective of our quest. Finally emerges Lord Dhanvantari—the bearer of the *amrit*—which can bestow life immortal beyond the confines of this physical mortal frame!

As we meditate sincerely and consistently under the guidance of a realized guru, our consciousness moves upwards towards more refined stages and from a gross dark body we move on to a body of light. Christ said that the eye is the light of the body. If your eyes become single, that is to say if the current of attention is drawn back and focused at the third eye, your body will become refulgent or filled with light. 'The light of the body is the eye; if therefore thine eye be single, thy whole body shall be full of light' (Bible, Matthew 6:22).

Finally emerges Lord Dhanvantari—the bearer of the *amrit*—which can bestow life immortal beyond the confines of this physical mortal frame!

It is now that Lord Dhanvantari will manifest within us because, after all, he is also a manifestation of our higher Self. When we look at Lord Dhanvantari's image from this perspective, we realize that the pot which he holds is actually the multidimensional human body and the *amrit* which is contained therein is our true Self. Once the Self disentangles itself from the body and the mind, it shines in its own light, knowing it is deathless and hence, immortal—a spark of the same substance as the source,[21] ('So God created man in His own image; in the image of God He created him; male and female He created them.') with which it must merge to attain everlasting bliss of complete union, the summit of all yoga.

Notes

1. Rigvedic Maharishi Parashara, *The Vishnu Purana*, tr. H.H. Wilson, Creagte Space Independent Publishing Platform, 1840, p. 76.
2. Sardar Bahadur Maharaj Jagat Singh, 'The Science of the Soul', *Axioms of Spirituality*, Amritsar: Radha Soami Satsang Beas, 1952, p. 79.
3. Maharaj Sawan Singh, 'The Dawn of Light', *Prison House of Eighty-four*, Amritsar: Radha Soami Satsang Beas, 1985, p. 223.
4. Sardar Bahadur Maharaj Jagat Singh, 'The Science of the Soul', *The Wonderful House in Which We Live,* Amritsar: Radha Soami Satsang Beas, 1959, p. 39.
5. 'Finding Peace & Happiness at Last' on www.rssb.org, accessed June 2016, Maharaj Charan Singh, 'The Path', *The Living Master*, Amritsar: Radha Soami Satsang Beas, 2000, pp. 82–3.
6. 'A Spiritual Perspective' on www.rssb.org, accessed June 2016.
7. 'Running from Death, Longing for Love' on www.rssb.org, accessed June 2016; Maharaj Charan Singh, 'Die to Live', *Dying While Living,* Amritsar: Radha Soami Satsang Beas, 1999, p. 24.
8. J.C. Sethi, 'Santo Ki Bani', vol. I, Amritsar: Radha Soami Satsang Beas, 2012, pp. 184–5.
9. Revd Ebenezer Burgess, 'Translation of the Surya Siddhanta: A Textbook of Hindu Astronomy', *Of the Different Modes of Reckoning Time*, University of Calcutta, 1860, p. 319.
10. https://pparihar.com/2015/01/04/padma-puran-8-4-million-of-species-in-earth.
11. Maureen Lockhart, 'The Subtle Energy Body', *Theosophy, Anthroposophy, and the Subtle Bodies*, Vermont: Inner Traditions, 2010, pp. 154–5.
12. 'Atman is Distinct from the Pancha Koshas', on www.sivanandaonline.org, accessed June 2016; Shri Swami Sivananda, 'Kundalini Yoga', *Yoga & its Consummation*, The Divine Life Society, Sivanand Nagar, 1994, p. 127.
13. Ibid.
14. David Frawley, 'Yoga and Ayurveda', *The Soul & its different Bodies*, Wisconsin: Lotus Press, 1999, pp. 83–4. Susan G. Shumsky, 'Multidimensional Auric Field', *Exploring Auras*, Franklin Lakes, NJ: The Career Press, 2006, p. 65.
15. David Frawley, 'Yoga and Ayurveda', *The Soul & its different Bodies*, New Delhi: Lotus Press, 1999, p. 81.
16. Swami Rama, Rudolph Ballentine and Swami Ajaya, 'The Evolution of Consciousness—Yoga and Psychotherapy', *The Mind*, Honesdale, Pennsylvania: Himalayan International Institute of Yoga Science and Philosophy, 1976, p. 99.
17. Ibid.
18. Ibid.

19. Maharaj Sawan Singh, 'Philosophy of the Masters, vol. I', Amritsar: Radha Soami Satsang Beas, 1967, pp. xix–xx.
20. Maharaj Jagat Singh, 'The Science of the Soul', pp. 81–2.
21. Genesis-1:27 NKJV—The Bible.

References

Das, Lama Surya, *Tibetan Dream Yoga*, Boulder, CO: Sounds True, Inc., 2000.

Naimy, Mikhail, *The Book of Mirdad*, London: Watkins Publishing, 2002.

Rinpoche, Sogyal, *The Tibetan Book of Living and Dying*, Harper Collins Paperback, 1994.

Singh, Maharaj Charan, *Divine Light*, Amritsar: Radha Soami Satsang Beas, 1967.

———, *Santan Di Bani, Bani Sant Kabir Ji*, Amritsar: Radha Soami Satsang Beas, 1970.

Singh, Maharaj Sawan, *Philosophy of the Masters*, series IV, Amritsar: Radha Soami Satsang Beas, 1967.

Singh, Sardar Bahadur Jagat, *Discourses on Sant Mat*, vol. II, Amritsar: Radha Soami Satsang Beas, 2006.

Sivananda, Swami, *Atman is Distinct from the Pancha Koshas*, The Divine Life Society, 2011.

2

Anatomy in
Diverse Schools

T.I. RADHAKRISHNAN

ACCORDING TO MODERN MEDICINE, anatomy is the study of the structure of the body. It is studied as a structural, embryological and histological concept. Structural anatomy in modern medicine includes musculoskeletal, vascular, nervous, digestive, respiratory, genitourinary and sense systems. From the medical point of view, surgical anatomy has made great progress in the twentieth and twenty-first centuries. These two centuries are also the centuries of transplantation. For example, in 1964, Dr Christian Barnard performed the world's first heart transplant. All kinds of transplants have been done, except that of the brain which was done in the Vedas.

Anatomy has also been studied in Ayurveda. According to it, the body is made up of *panchabhutas* (elements)—*prithvi, tej, jal, vayu* and *akash* and are represented in the three forces—*vata, pitta* and *kapha*. These *panchabhutas* arose from the *triguna* or atom. An atom has positrons, neutrons and electrons. When charged positively, it is called the positron or *rajoguna*. When charged negatively, it is called the electron or *tamoguna* and when in neutral form, it is called *sattvaguna*.

The *triguna* from *ahankar* (feeling of self) arises from *mahat,* i.e. cosmic intellect. *Mahat* arises from *avyakta*—a concealed form of pure existence—which arises from uncertainty or non-existence.

In the Ayurvedic principle of anatomy, one should understand philosophical principles such as *Nyaya-Vaisheshika, Sankhya, Mimamsa,* Yoga and Vedanta. Of these, the first three systems are more important.

Vaisheshika starts from the creation of the universe. In the *Vaisheshika Siddhantha*, we have the atomic theory of Kanada, who says that the atom is not divisible. The modern scientists were of the same belief. It is only now that we know atoms can be divided into many subatomic particles. But note that Adi Sankara in the *Brahma Sutra* clearly said that the atom can be divided.

There are three words we should know when we study Ayurvedic anatomy. They are *purusha, sharir* and *shayrir*. While *sharir* denotes only anatomy, *shayrir* implies anatomy with its physiology. Ayurveda also has the *dhatu* systems—*rasadhatu* (plasma), *mansam* (muscle), *metha* (fat), *majja* (marrow), *shukra* (semen), *rakta* (blood) and *asthi* (bone). Ayurveda discusses anatomy in detail, just as modern anatomy does. However, unlike in Ayurveda, modern anatomy *dissects* and studies the body, which is quite helpful from a surgical point of view. In Ayurveda, embryology is called *garbha-sharir* and has details of the development of the embryo into a baby for every month. In Homoeopathy too, we have the study of anatomy and physiology, and the body is dissected as in modern medicine.

In Acupuncture, the Chinese system of medicine, one must know anatomy very well as only then will one know actual acupuncture points such as the nerve plexuses, nerve centres and nerve endings of the body. In Kerala, there is a system of acupuncture called the *Marma* and the *Kalari* system. The difference between this and the Chinese system is that while the latter uses a metallic needle, in *Marma* and *Kalari*, a biological needle—the thumb—is used to press points. That is important because humans are biological creatures and therefore a biological method is more useful and practical from the medical point of view.

Coming to Yoga, there are six *chakras* which have their effects on anatomy. While all six are in the form of a *chakra*, the *sahasrarapadma* is not. *Sahasrarapadma* is the crowning *chakra* which controls everything in the body. *Chakras* have a direct link with modern anatomy. *Chakras* are the nerve plexuses of the autonomic nervous system. For example, when one has had food, it goes to the intestines and changes to waste without one's knowledge. The same goes for the heart which beats at 72 beats per minute. So, the *chakras* have a physical as well as an energy basis. Though most yogis say that they are all energy *sandesh* with no physical basis, this cannot be true. *Chakras* have a physical as well as a metaphysical existence. The *manipura chakra*, for example, has 10 petals and these correspond with the solar plexus which has 10 branches. So is the case with *Marma* which is said to be 107 in the body. These are nerve plexuses and if stimulated, one gets good results.

To conclude, we must realize that our biography is our biology. We all have immense powers of healing in us and only we can become our own doctors. In order to become the best doctor, we must control the functioning of the autonomic nervous system. Until then, we cannot become yogis. Let this be the anatomy for the next century.

References

FOR ANATOMY IN VARIOUS SYSTEMS OF MEDICINE

1. Gray Henry, *Gray's anatomy*, originally published 1858.
2. Professor Thatte D.G., *Sharira Rachana Vigyan*.
3. *Charaka Samhita*.
4. *Sushruta Samhita*.
5. *Marmachikitsa*.

FOR MIND AND DISEASES

1. Interview, Max Plank with J.W.N. Sullivan, in *The Observer*, 1931.
2. Lipton Bruce, *Biology of Belief*.
3. Lloyd Alex, *Healing Code*.
4. *Charaka Samhita*.
5. *Mandukya Upanishad*.
6. *Rigveda*.

3

The Supra-Physical Anatomy of Unani Medicine is the Basis of its Past and Present Holism

K.M.Y. AMIN

U NANI ANATOMY, INDEED ANATOMY of all traditional medicines, is radically different from its modern conception. It will be difficult, if not impossible, for contemporary minds to even broadly understand the anatomy of traditional medicines. Unani anatomy, like the anatomy of all traditional medicines, describes not only the body structure, which is the entirety of modern anatomy, but also the supra-physical dimensions of the human being. This is so because traditional medicines have a vision of the entirety of being, of which the physical part is only a tiny fragment, like the proverbial tip of the iceberg showing above the water surface.

So, first, Unani anatomy includes an elaborate description of body structure, both analytic and synthetic, but much more remarkably, it encompasses the supra-physical roots of the body also. Second, it possesses observable indicators of these supra-physical roots so that an ordinary human being, not blessed by higher vision, can also apprehend the character of an individual's supra-physical level. For instance, dense, dark, thick and curly hair indicate hot, wet and sanguine temperament. However, the fact that human beings, comprising of physical and supra-physical levels, have an overall temperament and that it can be known by observable indicators, was originally discovered by sages having a higher consciousness. Empedocles (*c.*450 BC) is credited with describing the Four Elements.[1] He was a devotee of Orphic religion[2] which included exercises for activating higher consciousness. So, it is probable that he himself intuited these elements or learned them from earlier Orphic sages, probably via Pythagoreans.

It should be appreciated right at the outset that the remarkable holism and the resultant efficacy and safety of traditional medicines is the chief reason for their continuous though rather grudging use. This use is totally dependent upon their vision and use of the supra-physical roots of man.

Unani anatomy, though obscure for modern mentality, has the benefit of being supported by sister phenomena in other traditional medicines. But the particular Unani vision of the supra-physical roots and the method of diagnosing it is significantly different from other traditional medicines; the upshot being that the Unani schema is much easier to understand and practise in this age and day when the cosmos has become more opaque and the psyche of man less perspicacious. The advanced reader will be eager to know the reasons for this ease of practice of supra-physical based Unani health care, which should become clear towards the end of this essay.

Here it suffices to say that Providence joined the particular type of philosophization appearing in Greece to a new mode of Revelation, i.e. Islam. Greek philosophy represented, so to speak, the Substance or *Prakriti* of the Last Times, while Islam was the contemporary expression of *Purusha*, that could allow natural sciences to emerge, which were positivistic and objective, like Western science, but unlike it, took into account at least the subtle, if not the spiritual, roots of corporeal objects. Such sciences, like Unani medicine, were holistic unlike Western reductionist sciences. At the same time, unlike the more ancient and subjective traditional sciences, these Graeco-Islamic sciences were more comprehensible for the intuitionally attenuated and observationally inclined people of these murky Last Times called *Qurb-e-Qayamat* in Islam and *Kaliyuga* in Hinduism. More importantly, these positivistic but trans-physical sciences continued to provide openings to the supra-corporeal level of Reality and, thus, helped rather than hindered the realization of the Absolute (*Tawhid/Moksha*).

The peculiar ease of apprehending the supra-physical roots of man in Unani medicine depends upon the Greek cosmology on which it rests. In the seventh century, Muslims conquered two great seats of ancient learning, Jundishapur founded in third century CE in Iran by Sassanian Emperor Shapur and Alexandria, founded by Alexander in third century BC. They translated the ancient learning and medicine of Greece, Egypt, Mesopotamia, Iran, China and India available in these centres into

Arabic in the seventh–ninth centuries. Although they benefited from the learning of all civilizations, they based their sciences on Greek learning and cosmology. Ali Bin Sahl Rabban Tabari (*c*.850 CE), who was proficient in Greek and Syriac, drew upon this corpus to write the first major text of Unani medicine based upon Greek cosmology and medicine. But his knowledge of other cosmologies and medicines is shown by the inclusion of a long appendix on Indian medicine in the book entitled, *Firdaws al Hikmah fi al Tib* (Paradise of Wisdom in Medicine).[3] Although Muslims were aware of other ancient cosmologies too, they based their learning on Greek cosmology. However, it should be maintained right from the beginning that this cosmology was appropriated selectively and was systematized and modified to get it in line with Islam's Unitary and transcendental vision.

The key to understand the distinct character of this cosmology is its simplicity. The entire universe is made up of only four elements: air, fire, water and earth. These elements are characterized by only one set of four qualities (*kaifiyat*), i.e. hot or cold and dry or wet. Thus, air is hot and wet, fire is hot and dry, earth is cold and dry and water is cold and wet. Each entity is formed by the dynamic mixing and interaction of elements and their overall character, called *mizaj* (temperament). So, each man is hot and dry or hot and wet or cold and dry or cold and wet. Similarly, each drug, diet or environmental factor is also hot and dry or hot and wet or cold and dry or cold and wet. Hence the mind-boggling simplicity of Graeco-Islamic cosmology in describing the basic character or supra-physical root of each individual member, and of all the coordinates of health care, by only four qualities.

The discerning reader would have appreciated that this simplicity lies not only in the small number of these parameters but also in the complete integration of the scheme as the *same parameters are used for describing all coordinates*. An important detail to be noted is that according to Greek cosmology, particularly as elaborated by Aristotle, the immediate substrata of man and animate entities are the four humours (*akhlat*, singular: *khilt*)—blood (*dam*), phlegm (*balgham*), yellow bile (*safrah*) and black bile (*sawdah*). Thus, the overall character or *mizaj* of a man is commonly described in terms of the preponderant humour. However, as each humour corresponds to a particular element and, thereby, to the qualities of this element, *mizaj* can be translated in terms of the qualities rather than the humours.

Since the *mizaj* of inanimate coordinates of health care—drug, diet and environmental factors—are described in terms of qualities, they can be easily correlated with the overall character of man by translating the humoural *mizaj* into the qualitative *mizaj*. Thus, the parallel description of man in humoural terms does not detract from the simplicity of describing all coordinates of health care on the basis of the same four qualities, i.e. hot or cold and dry or wet.

This simplicity can be better appreciated by comparison with Ayurveda where man is described by three *doshas* made from five *mahabhutas*, while drugs are described by six *rasas* constituted by five *mahabhutas*. Further, *mahabhutas*, and the *doshas* and *rasas* arising from them, are only physical (*bhautik*) and, therefore, do not describe the whole man. His subtle level (*sukshma sharir*) is described by a separate set of parameters, mainly consisting of *gunas*.

Thus, Ayurveda and its chief underlying cosmology, namely, *Sankhya Darshan*, are more complex and relatively difficult to master as they describe the physical and subtle level of man by two different sets of elements, namely, *mahabhutas* and *tanmatras*, respectively, whereas, drugs are described by other sets of referents, mainly the *rasas*. The Greek cosmology and Unani medicine, on the contrary, describe both the physical and subtle level of man, drug, diet, etc., by a common set of Four Elements and their Four Qualities (*Kaifiyat*). However, if the simplicity of Unani medicine makes it more comprehensible in these times, the complexity of Ayurveda gives to it a distinct ancient richness, e.g. its ability to conceive and use not only concrete things like drugs, but also the modification of higher consciousness as a means of health care, by creating space within its scheme of medicine for the semi-scientific and semi-religious sister discipline of Yoga. On the other hand, Unani medicine alludes to higher consciousness as a factor of health care in more muted and totally religious (and not scientific) terms, by only inchoately suggesting the positive role of religious beliefs and practices. This reticence is probably due to the simpler cosmological schema of Unani medicine. It should be remembered that here utilization of higher consciousness is under consideration, not psychotherapy, which Unani medicine possesses in a good measure.

The second dimension of the simplicity of this cosmology is that the parameters used are easy to understand intellectually as well as for practical measurements. First, these essentially supra-physical qualities have clear physical or sensible extensions, i.e. everyone can feel them on one's fingertips. Second, other physical and sensible expressions of these qualities—for example, thick, curly, and dark hair indicating heat and their opposite types indicating cold—are also easy to figure out and seem to be connected to these qualities even by common sense.

The third, and very profound, dimension of the simplicity of Graeco-Islamic cosmology is that the same few parameters, i.e. the four qualities, are used for describing *all levels of Being*. For instance, both the physical body (*aza*) and the subtle *pneuma* (*arwah*, singular: *ruh*) of man are fully described by these four qualities. This becomes possible because the same four elements (*arkan*) are seen to make up not only the physical or corporeal body but also the subtle *pneuma*. In Ayurveda, however, the elements (*mahabhutas*) are corporeal in nature and only make up the physical body (*dosha* or *dhatu*), the subtle components of man (*prana, tejas, ojas*, etc.) being made up of other substances arising from the five *tanmatras*.

Thus, the fact that the same four elements make up both the physical as well as the subtle level of man, drug, diet, etc., allows Unani medicine to use the four qualities of these four elements to describe and correlate not only the overall character of the physical level but also the overall character of the subtle level.

The Mind-Body Unity in Unani Medicine

Unani medicine substantializes the mind because it considers psychic *pneuma* (*ruf nafsani*) to be the substance of the mind. This psychic *pneuma*, being made up of the subtle form of the four elements (*arkan*) can be described in terms of the very same four qualities, which are used for describing the body (*aza*). Thus, depression, arising due to increase of the subtle form of the humour black bile, cold and dry, in psychic *pneuma*, can be diagnosed by physical and psychic symptoms of coldness and dryness, and can be treated by giving drugs having opposite qualities, i.e. hotness and wetness. This shows that the simplicity of Unani medicine's schema of supra-physical roots, characterized in this case by its vision of essentially supra-physical four elements, allows it to effectively unify both the mind and the body, and describe both the psychic and somatic dimensions of man by the same set of symptoms of the four qualities of the elements.

Starting with Descartes, modern Western philosophy contrasts the mind with the body, implying an association of consciousness with corporeality and of movement or power with corporeality. All other traditional philosophies contrast the mind with other functions like movement, etc., but not with the body. This is so because not only the mind, but all other systems or functions of the body, like movement, growth, etc., are subservient to both bodily and other subtle matrices. Thus, in Unani medicine, just as the mental function is served by the subtle psychic *pneuma*, with its seat in the brain, similarly, the metabolic and nutritional function is served by an equally subtle natural *pneuma* (*ruh tabii*) having its seat in the liver. So, according to traditional medicines, mind is not the only subtle organ; all organs have a subtle extension.

It should be appreciated that Unani medicine effectively unifies mind and body by substantializing the mind which amounts to describing its structure in a substantial, rather than merely diagrammatic manner. The essentially supra-physical elements of Unani medicine, which develop physicality or corporeality in the lower reaches of their mixed state, allow Unani medicine to visualize even a supra-physical substance, and to apprehend both the subtle substance of the *pneuma* and the gross substance of the body by means of quality-based symptoms. On the other hand, Ayurveda visualizes the mind mainly in terms of its functions, i.e. the sensory and motor organs (*indriyas*). Since Western medicine conceives the mind as an effect or property of brain molecules, so it can be considered to molecularize the mind. In comparison, like Ayurveda, Unani medicine conceives the mind as an actual thing rather than mere property or epiphenomenon, thereby possessing a well-developed psychiatric and psychosomatic medicine. By substantializing the mind, Unani becomes more objective, precise and easy to practise. However, because its mental substance is subtle and not reduced to only physical molecules, its psychiatry and psychosomatic medicine is much wider and satisfactory.

The Unitary vision of Islam helped Unani medicine to unify the mind and the body more effectively. It did so by adopting the supra-physical Greek elements which provide a common substantial basis to both mind and body, rather than the corporeal *mahabhutas*, which lie behind the body while indicating the substance of the *manas*—only sketchily and indirectly—by the three *gunas*. The Unitarian preference for principles that lie behind maximum levels and modes of reality provides part of the explanation for the Muslims' intriguing historical choice of Greek cosmology.

Unani Medicine fully extended the implicit logic of original Greek medicine, to clearly describe the mind as a substance, and manipulate it by using other substances such as drugs. Unani medicine views the mind as the sum of psychic faculty (mental function) and psychic *pneuma* (mental substance). But it approaches and manipulates the mind mainly in terms of the psychic *pneuma*. As shown earlier, this substantialization makes Unani psychiatry objective and precise like psychiatry in Western medicine. Just as the understanding of the transcendental principle in

Islamic metaphysics becomes easier for the less intuitive modern mind when viewed as the object, similarly, the substantialization of mind makes the understanding and manipulation of mind easier in Unani psychiatry and psychosomatic medicine.

The subject and the object are the two poles of reality here. Though metaphysics can emphasize one pole, it cannot totally ignore the other one. So, Islamic metaphysics, despite describing reality in the objective mode as Being,[4] also briefly refers to it as Consciousness.

Consciousness and Unani Medicine

Unani medicine uses consciousness as a minor determinant of psychic health, by means of suggestive psychotherapy and recommends religious counselling. However, as explained earlier, it uses the substance of mind and its manipulation by pharmacotherapy and drugs, as the major determinant of psychiatric health care.

Unani medicine though technically limited to the subtle and physical substance of man, does provide space for the spiritual dimension while handing it over to the religious sector. In fact, most Unani physicians were simultaneously devout and spiritual people who also provided spiritual counselling while practising the narrower technical Unani medicine. In pre-modern India, and to some extent even today, many eminent Sufis and *ulama* (religious scholars) practised Unani medicine.[5] On the other hand, many Unani physicians were disciples of Sufi Masters. The term *Tib al Nabawi* (prophetic medicine) has sometimes been used to cover the spiritual dimension of medicine in the Islamic civilization.

Holism

Traditional medicine's schema of the supra-physical root of man, drug, etc., is no mere academic trivia but the essential basis of their most valuable and unique character, which is Holism. It is necessary to discuss holism, its remarkable advantages and the reason why it becomes possible only by using the vision of traditional medicines and the supra-physical root or substratum of man, drug, etc.

Holism means the ability to describe the overall character of a man, disease, drug, diet, etc. The tremendous benefit of knowing the overall character of a disease and drug is the consequent possibility of fully matching a disease with a drug of the opposite type. This contrast matching ensures full removal or radical cure of a disease, obviating residual symptoms and relapses, as well as the absence of tangential swings of the patient's physiology or overshooting adverse effects when the influence of the drug ends.

The apprehension of this holistic or overall character becomes possible by addressing an entity, for example, a man, at the supra-physical level, particularly at the lowest stratum of the supra-physical level, i.e. the subtle level. Supra-physical levels, including the subtle ones, are simple and can be apprehended as a whole or in profile, while the physical or corporeal level is complex and differentiated, and hence, not knowable as a whole. This difficulty in taking a holistic view becomes acute when going to the microscopic or molecular level of the physical stratum. That is why Western medicine does not succeed, and can never succeed in knowing the overall character of man, despite aspiring to it, because it limits itself only to the physical, and now, the molecular level of reality. It should be noted that systems biology, genomics and the bewildering array of all the 'omics' have not succeeded in making Western medicine holistic.

Correlation of Holistic Traditional Medicines and Biomolecular Western Medicine

The biomolecular Western medicine is so different, and apparently so advanced than traditional medicines, that the necessity of giving them a molecular dimension, if not a complete molecular makeover, appears to be almost an a priori truth. But nothing could be more patently wrong for the simple reason that traditional medicines enjoy the advantage of holism over Western medicine, precisely for the reason that they have certain principles and bases which Western medicine lacks.

So, the addition of Western medicine's molecular perspective to them needs to be done in a manner that does not violate the unique and traditional principles of these medicines, and thereby does not impair the existing benefits of these medicines. More importantly, we also need to discuss the degree of usefulness of molecular additions to traditional medicines, primary or secondary, and the exact areas where it will be of greater or lesser benefit to the existing powers of traditional medicines. For instance, botanical identification or determination of pesticidal contamination of traditional drugs would be of greater use, while determination of their molecular mechanism of action would produce only modest increase in their usefulness and that too not with all types of drugs.

So, in light of the impermissibility of a blanket molecularization, we should identify the principles for determining the limited areas of correlation of traditional and Western medicine. One such principle can be derived from the above discussion of holism. Since the valuable and remarkable holism of traditional medicines depends upon their schemas of supra-physical roots—such as *mizaj*, in the case of Unani medicine, these medicines should be practised primarily on the basis of these schemas, and molecular effects should be used, if at all, only secondarily. For instance, depression should be basically visualized as a cold and dry disease to be treated by hot and wet drugs. However, tentative shortlisting can secondarily be done by selecting those hot and wet drugs which may be increasing brain monoamines, as depression is associated with their reduction. Thus, the primary basis of conceiving disease (pathology) and treatment (therapeutics) should be the traditional schema of supra-physical roots, i.e. *mizaj* in the case of Unani medicine and *dosha-rasa* in the case of Ayurveda. It is irrational to translate these schemas into molecular terms for the simple reason that they basically describe the supra-physical level of man, whereas molecules pertain only to the physical level. It is also not justified to replace the traditional clinical signs and symptoms by molecular tests for diagnosing the supra-physical *mizaj*, *prakriti*, etc., the reason being that these phenomena are holistic, are better diagnosed by clinical parameters which too are holistic rather than by molecules, which are fragmentary and reductive. However, once the disease and its treatment has been identified in terms of *mizaj* or *dosha-rasa*, further fine-tuning may be done with the help of molecular biology.

Conclusion

Traditional medicines should be understood in the supra-physical and physical perspective rather than in merely physical (molecular) perspective. Since, the latter has largely happened till now, traditional medicines require rediscovery of their actual traditional character more than research for their optimal utilization. A blanket modernization, which effectively means molecularization, will do away with their supra-physical principles like *mizaj*, *dosha-rasa*, etc., and thereby remove their remarkable and unmatched quality of holism which completely depends upon these schemas.

But modernization in some limited areas may be of benefit, like in the botanical identification of drugs or in short-listing treatment on the basis of molecular effects after selecting the drugs primarily on the basis of supra-physical schemas like *mizaj*, *guna-rasa*, etc. So, guiding principles should be developed for identifying the beneficial from harmful modernization.

The distinctive trans-physical Unani schema is based on the unique character of Islamic metaphysics which describes reality mainly in the object mode as Being, rather than in the subject mode as Consciousness, and adopts a preeminently Unitarian perspective. That is why it appropriated Greek cosmology which describes the physical or corporeal level as well as the subtle level of Being. (Hindu cosmology, on the other hand, describes two different substrata for the corporeal and subtle level, i.e. *mahabhutas* and *gunas* respectively.)

Thus, with the help of a Unitarian vision and a Greek cosmology which integrated the physical and subtle levels, the Arabs built a simple and substantialized schema of supra-physical root common to all health care correlates that allow access to supra-physical roots, hence paving the way for holism, even for the intuitionally attenuated modern man.

One important part accruing from the unique unitarianism and substantialization of Unani medicine is an objective but subtle psychiatry based upon the drug treatment of the subtle mental substance without reducing the mind to mere molecules, *à la* Western medicine. Galen (b. 130 CE) denoted the subtle level of man by *pneuma* (Arabic: *ruh*) but owing to the increasing materialization of Greek mind, he did not give it any physiological role. By the time of Ibn Sina (b. 980 CE), the Muslim expropriators of this medicine made *pneuma* a well-defined subtle substance arising from the humours, not only subsuming the brain as mind (cf. *Manomaya Kosh*), but also subsuming the rest of the body and organs, as the vital principle (cf. *Pranamaya Kosh*).[6] Being substantialized and derived from the humours, all humour-led pharmacotherapy became applicable to the *pneumatic* mind and its psychiatric diseases. Being derived from the subtle components of humours, it provided an independent subtle ontology to mental phenomena, thus preventing their materialistic reduction and obscuration.

Thus, Unani medicine is based on pharmacotherapy, and hence includes an easy to practise psychiatry, which is quite adequate to the subtle and supra-physical nature of the mind.

In addition to being approached as a subtle substance, the mind is also addressed as Consciousness. But, consciousness based interventions are handed over to Islam and its esoteric dimension—*Tasawwuf* (Sufism), just as Ayurveda hands it over to Dharma and Yoga, the difference lying not so much in Ayurveda but in Hinduism, where esoterism (Yoga) is overtly accepted and its scientific dimension is well defined.

The traditional schema of supra-physical roots are very crucial to the powers and plus points of traditional medicines and they can be understood only if one has both the supra-physical and physical worldviews. Because modern minds are mainly physically oriented, traditional medicines have been poorly understood or misunderstood. So, they have to be, in a sense, rediscovered, by very precise study.

Since the celebrated holism of traditional medicines is dependent on their schemas of the supra-physical root of man, no attempt should be made to replace the *mizaj* or *dosha-rasa* based pathology and pharmacology by their Western medicine molecular versions. To spotlight the utter impossibility of having a holistic medicine on the basis of molecular pathology and pharmacology, one should appreciate that molecule-based attempts at holism like systems biology, genomics, proteomics, etc., are illogical and practically unsuccessful.

Second, since supra-physical based overall characters, like *mizaj* or *prakriti* are holistic and subjective phenomena, holistic physical parameters—clinical signs and symptoms—are more suited to diagnose them. Contemporary experience of traditional physicians reveals that these classical signs and symptoms help in diagnosing *mizaj* and others quite easily with sufficient precision. So, it is not that only *mizaj*, etc., should not be replaced by molecular systems, even the traditional clinical signs and symptoms prescribed for diagnosing them should not be replaced by molecular parameters.

However, the application of modern techniques and approaches in some limited areas can have very significant to moderately significant role in the optimization of traditional medicines. But the small areas of application and the type of application should be rigorously defined to avoid inappropriate and harmful use of modern science. Although, modern science and modern research does have a role in the optimization of traditional medicines, but rediscovery, as delineated above, is more crucial to their optimization.

Unani medicine's specific, unified and substantialized schema of supra-physical roots of man, drug, etc., and the unique advantages that it confers on Unani medicine should be recognized and appreciated.

Notes

1. S.H. Nasr, *Science and Civilization in Islam*, Cambridge, Mass.: Harvard University Press, 1968, p. 219.
2. Bertrand Russell, *History of Western Philosophy*, London: George Allen & Unwin, 1961, pp. 71–5.
3. Nasr, *Science and Civilization in Islam*, p. 196.

4. Although in the *mashshai* (peripatetic) sector of Islamic philosophy, *wujud* is Being in the usual sense, but in integral Islamic philosophy, particularly the *irfani* (gnostic) sector, *wujud*, paradoxically, also covers what is otherwise called Non-Being, Beyond-Being or Godhead.
5. Fabrizio Speziale, Newsletter of Institute of Asian Studies, Leiden, no. 30, <www.iias.nl/> accessed March 2003.
6. M. Ullman, *Islamic Medicine*, Edinburgh University Press, 1978, pp. 61–3.

References

Coomaraswamy, A.K., *A New Approach to the Vedas: An Essay in Translation and Exegesis*, New Delhi: Munshiram Manoharlal, 2002.

Dash, V.B., *Fundamentals of Ayurvedic Medicine*, Delhi: Indian Books Centre, 1999.

Guénon, R., *Introduction to the Study of Oriental Doctrines*, Lahore: Suhail Academy, 2011.

Nasr, S.H., *Islamic Philosophy from its Origin to the Present*, State University of New York Press, 2006.

———, *Science and Civilization in Islam*, Cambridge, Mass.: Harvard University Press, 1968.

Schuon, F., 'The Five Divine Presences', in *Dimensions of Islam*, London: George Allen & Unwin, 1970.

Ullman, M., *Islamic Medicine*, Edinburgh University Press, 1978.

4

Udal Thathuvam

Physiology of Siddha System of Medicine

R.S. RAMASWAMY

T HE SIDDHA SYSTEM OF MEDICINE, one of the major Indian systems of medicine, is widely practised in south India, especially in Tamil Nadu, Kerala and Puducherry. It is also popular in Sri Lanka, Malaysia and Singapore where considerable number of Tamilians live. It is a very ancient system of medicine and its origin dates back to 3000 BC.

The originator of this system is said to be Shiva, who preached it to his consort Parvathy, who, in turn, preached it to Nandhidevar. Then, Nandhidevar preached it to Agathiyar, who then passed it on to other Siddhars. This system was traditionally handed down in the form of verses. They were initially in the oral tradition, then written on palm leaf manuscripts and later, printed in books.

Medicine becomes indispensable when diseases affect the body, mind and soul. In *Thirumanthiram*, Siddhar Thirumoolar defines Siddha as:

One that cures a physical ailment is medicine
One that prevents ailment is medicine and
One that bestows immortality is medicine.

Unlike other modern medical systems, Siddha aims not only to cure diseases of the body and the mind, but also those of the soul, by purification which leads to salvation. The last line of the above verse indicates that Siddha is also for spiritual health.

Udal Thathuvam: Physiology

In Siddha, *Udal Thathuvam* means 'truths or principles related to the human body'. *Adippadai Thathuvam* means 'basic principle'. The 96 *thathuvams* described by Siddhar Yugi are all scientific and unchallengeable, because the principles are irrefutable and applicable even today. The principles are agreeable to modern science also.

An important Siddha principle is, 'Existence will never go and non-existence will never come.' Siddha thus brings out the analogy between *andam* (the Universe) and *pindam* (the human body). The view that whatever is found in the universe is also found in the human body is explained in the Siddha book *Sattamuni Gnanam*. In fact, there is a relationship between planets and organs too as listed below:

Heart—Sun (*Gnayiru*)
Brain—Moon (*Thingal*)
Gall bladder—Mars (*Sevvai*)
Lungs—Mercury (*Buthan*)
Liver—Jupiter (*Guru*)
Kidneys—Venus (*Sukkiran*)
Spleen—Saturn (*Sani*)

96 Principles

Siddha has 96 principles which can be further subdivided.

THE FIRST SET OF PRINCIPLES—*ANMA THATHUVAM*

These are 30 and are related to the soul:

Panchabutham (five elements)—5
Pori (sense organs)—5
Pulan (senses)—5
Kanmenthiriyam (organs of motor action)—5
Gnanenthiriyam (organs of perception)—5
Karanam (intellectual faculties)—4
Arivu (knowledge)—1

Panchabutham or five elements constitute the universe as well as man. They are: *mann* (earth), *neer* (water), *thee* (fire), *vali/katru* (air) and *veli* (space/ether). *Porigal* or five sense organs constitute: *mei* (skin), *vai* (mouth, i.e. the tongue), *kann* (eye), *mookku* (nose) and *sevi* (ear). *Pulangal* are the five senses and they comprise of: *suvai* (taste), *oli* (vision), *ooru* (touch), *osai* (hearing) and *natram* (smell). The *panchabutham* are related to the *pulangal* in this way: *suvai*—water, *oli*—fire, *ooru*—air, *osai*—space/ether and *natram*—earth.

Man also possesses a sixth sense. *Tholkappium*, the earliest book on Tamil grammar and literature, writes, *Mavum Makkalum Iyarivinave Makkal thame ararivuyire*, which means that man differs from and is superior to other living beings by possession of his sixth sense, i.e. the power of reasoning, with which he can refrain from committing sins and lead a disciplined life. By this he can achieve salvation—the real end of human birth.

Further, Thiruvalluvar, the author of *Tirukkural*, a treatise on ethical principles, says, *Suvai oli ooru osai natram endru ainthin Vahai therivan katte ulagu*, which means that this world is functioning only with the knowledge of those capable of working, i.e. applying, the five senses sensibly. On control or withdrawal of the five senses, Siddhar Pathirakriyaar says, *Aangaram ulladakki aimpulanai chuttaruthu Thoongamal thoongi sugam peruvathu ekkalam* which means 'Subdue your ego, burn your five senses and get deeply absorbed in meditation till you reach the stage of self-realization'.

There are five organs of action, *kanmenthiriyangal*, which are: *vai* (mouth)—speech, *kal* (leg)—locomotion, *kai* (hand)—giving or receiving, *eruvai* (anal orifice)—defecation and *karuvai* (vaginal orifice)—parturition. The five organs of perception, *gnanenthiriyangal*, mediate the function of the senses through the sense organs. They constitute various parts of the nervous system which are responsible for the perception of the senses through the sense organs. This is how they mediate: the *mei* (skin) works in association with air and perceives tactile sensations, i.e. touch, pain and temperature. *Vai* (mouth, i.e. the tongue) mediates with water and perceives the sense of taste, *kann* (eye) works with fire to perceive the sense of vision, *mookku* (nose) works with earth and perceives the sense of smell and *sevi* (ear) mediates with space or ether and perceives the sense of hearing.

Anthakaranangal, the four inner organs or intellectual faculties are: *manam* which is responsible for thinking of an entity or simply a 'thought', *buddhi* which analyses the thought, *siddham*, which after analysis, takes a decision on whether to act or not and *ahangaram* which executes the decision of *siddham*.

Arivu literally means knowledge or knowing of one's self, i.e. *anma* or soul. It is linked to the life force. According to Thirumoolar's *Thirumanthiram* ('Siddha Maruthuvanga Churukkam'), the size of the life force can be illustrated like this: 'Take out a single hair of the cow and divide it into 100 parts. Take one among the 100 parts and divide it into 1,000. Then take one among those 1,000 parts and divide it into 1,00,000 parts and the size of one part among these is the size of the life-force.'

THE SECOND SET OF PRINCIPLES

Naadi—10
Vayu—10
Vidayam—5
Kosam—5

Naadi

In *naadigal* (*dasa naadis*), there are ten nerves or arteries of the human body which form channels for the flow of vital spirit. These are:

Idakalai: It originates from the right big toe and terminates into the left nostril.
Pinkalai: It originates from the left big toe and like a pair of scissors, terminates into the right nostril (decussation).
Suzhimunai (*Suzhumunai*): It starts from the *moolaadhaaram*, the base of the spinal cord, traverses up to the skull and forms the central base for all the other *naadis*.
Siguvai: It is located in the inner tongue and helps in swallowing (deglutition).
Purudan: It is located in the right eye (vision).
Kanthari: It is located in the left eye (vision).
Aththi: It is located in the right ear (hearing).
Alampudai: It is located in the left ear (hearing).
Sangini: It is located in the urethral or vaginal orifice (micturition, menstruation and parturition).
Guhu: It is located in the anal orifice (defecation).

Then, there is the *naadi* (pulse), the force responsible for the existence of life. Their combinations are as follows:

Idakalai + Abanan = Vali naadi (16 inches)
Pinkalai + Piranan = Azhal naadi (12 inches)
Suzhimunai + Samanan = Iya naadi (equal distribution)
Vatham : Pitham : Kabam = 1 : ½ : ¼

Other *naadis* include:

Bootha naadi: It is felt by the thumb and little finger to confirm the state of *kaya siddhi* (immortality), i.e. preparing for the *samadhi* state.
Guru naadi: It is felt beyond V, P and K (*vatham, pitham* and *kabam*). It influences

all other *naadis* and makes them function. It can exist in all the five *avathai* (states) of the soul. Changes in V, P and K will reflect in *guru naadi,* which in a complete sleepy state indicates death.

Vayu

Vayu (vital air) is also called *vali* or *kal* in Tamil and is divided into ten depending upon its locations and functions. It is said that the ten *vayus* support the functions of the ten *naadis.* These are:

1. *Praanan*: Originates from the centre of the skull
    Helps in inspiration, expiration and digestion
    Controls respiratory organs and maintains their functions
    Also called *uyirkkal,* meaning the *vayu* that nourishes the life force

2. *Apaanan*: Originates from the *mooladharam*
    Helps in assimilation of foodstuff after digestion and absorption
    Helps in urination, defecation
    Discharges semen, expulses ovum
    Expels the baby from the womb during delivery
    Acts through the anterior horn cells
    Also called *Keezh Nokkum Kaal,* meaning the *vayu* that acts with downward force

3. *Viyaanan*: Originating from the skin, it spreads all over the body
    Maintains circulation, ventilation, thermoregulation
    Perceives sensation through the skin
    Performs movements of both movable and immovable parts of the body
    Also called *paravukal,* meaning the *vayu* that acts by spreading the force all over the body

4. *Udhaanan*: Emanates from the fire of the stomach
    Resides in navel, neck (throat) and nose
    Mixes with the essence of digested foodstuff and reaches them to the required tissues (aids gastrointestinal motility)
    Responsible for the production of speech (vocal chords)
    Responsible for reflexes like cough, sneeze, hiccup and vomiting
    Establishes a link between stimulations from the external world and cerebral nerves (orientation)
    Acts from the cerebello-spinal junction (coordination)
    Also called *mel nokkumkal,* meaning the *vayu* that acts with upward force

5. *Samaanan*: Originates from the navel region
    Controls all other *vayus*
    Balances the six tastes, water and foodstuff during the process of digestion and reaches them to their sites of action
    Acts through the nerves, supplying gastrointestinal organs—mouth, esophagus, stomach, small intestine, large intestine, rectum and anus

Also called *nadukkal,* meaning the *vayu* that acts as a central force controlling the actions of other *vayus*

6. *Naagan:* Located in the white matter of the brain (esp. frontal lobe)
    Acts as an instrument for *anthakaranam*
    Responsible for one's intelligence, it activates the brain to learn all kinds of arts and to sing good songs
    Responsible for blinking and hair-raising (in alarming situations)

7. *Koorman:* Emanates from the *manam* (the mind)
    Acts on the eyes and produces blinking
    Responsible for the acts of yawning and closing of the mouth
    Acts through the facial nerve

8. *Kirukaran:* Acts on the tongue to produce salivary secretion and on the nose to produce nasal (mucous) secretion (Autonomic Nervous System, Cranial Nerve)
    Produces hunger
    Causes thinking of one entity
    Produces sneeze and cough
    Acts through the trigeminal and vagus nerves

9. *Devathathan:* Emanating in the form of a circle, it produces laziness and tiredness on waking up
    Causes the movements of the eyeball (3rd, 4th and 6th cranial nerves)
    Causes one to be engaged in coaxing, fighting, wordy quarrel and bouts of intense anger
    Resides in the rectum and genitalia
    Acts through nerves that control the functions of the heart and lungs

10. *Thananjeyan:* It swells up from the nose and causes swelling all over the body
    Produces a noise in the ear like that of the sea
    Gets expelled three days after death when the skull bursts open, after all the other gases are expelled from the body
    Post-mortem changes
    Acts on the skull-bone sinuses

Vidayam (Asayam—5)

1. *Iraikudal (Amarvasayam):* The site where the swallowed foodstuff stays, i.e. the stomach.
2. *Serikudal (Pahirvasayam):* The site where the foodstuff, after digestion, divides into nutritive essence and waste substances.
3. *Neerkkudal (Jalavasayam):* The site where the urine is formed, i.e. kidney, ureter and bladder.
4. *Malakkudal (Malavasayam):* The site where the faecal matter accumulates, i.e. the rectum.

5. *Venneerkkudal (Sukkilavasayam)*: The site where semen—*vindhu/natham* is formed, i.e. the testis/ovary.

Udambu (Kosam—5)

1. *Paruvudambu (Annamayakosam)*: The body constituted by the seven physical constituents, i.e. *saram, senneer* (blood), *oon* (flesh), *kozhuppu* (fat), *enbu* (bone), *moolai* (marrow/nervous tissue) and *sukkilam/suronitham* (sperm/ovum).
2. *Valiyudambu (Pranamayakosam)*: The body constituted by the combination of *pranan* and *kanmenthiriyam* (functional movements).
3. *Manavudambu (Manomayakosam)*: The body constituted by the *manam* and *gnanenthiriyam* (mental development, gaining knowledge and information).
4. *Arivudambu (Vignanamayakosam)*: The body constituted by the *buddhi* and *gnanenthiriyam* (gaining wisdom).
5. *Inbavudambu (Ananthamayakosam)*: The body constituted by the *pranavayu* and *suzhuthi* (a sleep-like state, blissful *samadhi* state).

THE THIRD SET OF PRINCIPLES

Atharam—6
Mandilam—3
Malam—3
Thodam—3
Edanai—3
Gunam—3
Vinai—2
Ragam—8
Avaththai—5

Atharam

There are six of them and they indicate the positions or levels through which the *kundalini shakthi* can be raised to reach the centre of perfection where the soul can realize God.

1. *Mooladharam*: It is located at the midpoint between the rectum and genital organ, i.e. at the base of the spinal cord. It is said to have influence over the sexual organs. It is here that the *kundalini shakthi* remains dormant.
2. *Swathishtanam*: It is located two finger breadths above the *mooladharam* in the navel region. It is said to have influence over the adrenal glands.
3. *Manipurakam*: It is located in the epigastric region, eight finger breadths above *Swathishtanam*. It forms the root of 1,008 blood vessels and nerves. It is said to have an influence over the pancreas.
4. *Anakatham*: It is located in the chest, ten finger breadths above *manipurakam*. It is said to have influence over the thymus gland.

5. *Visuddhi*: It is located in the throat region, ten finger breadths above *anakatham*. It is said to have influence over the thyroid gland.
6. *Ajnai*: It is located at the central point between the two eyebrows, twelve finger breadths above *visuddhi*. It is said to have influence over the pituitary gland.

Mandilam—3 (3 regions)

1. *Thee Mandilam (Agni mandilam)*: It is the region spreading from *mooladharam* to navel.
2. *Gnayiru Mandilam (Athithya mandilam)*: It is the region from *anakatham* to *visuddhi*.
3. *Thingal Mandilam (Chandra mandilam)*: It is located at the centre of the skull. It is called *amuthakalai*.

Malam—3

These are the attributes of the life force or soul:

1. *Anavam*: It is the egotism of an individual. *Anavam* is associated with the affinity towards worldly things.
2. *Mayai*: It is an entity which leads one to trouble by developing undue desires.
3. *Kanmam (Kamiyam)*: It means desire for everything. It leads one to commit good or bad deeds.

N.B.: Sweat, faeces and urine are *malams* related to the human body.

Thodam—3

The diseased or imbalanced condition of the *Uyir Thathu* (vital humour or vital life factor):

1. *Vatham (Vali)*: Derangement of *vayu* leading to disease.
2. *Pitham (Azhal)*: Derangement of *theyu* leading to disease.
3. *Kapham (Iyam)*: Derangement of (predominantly) *appu* leading to disease.

Edanai—3

It means desire or affinity, i.e. *patru*:

1. *Porul Patru*: It is the desire for material things.
2. *Puthalvar Patru*: It is the affinity or affection towards one's own children.
3. *Ulaga Patru*: It is the affinity or desire for the world and worldly things.

Gunam—3

It means quality:

1. *Saththuvam*: It is the possession of good qualities like humility, patience, truth, mercy, wisdom, love, self-control and austerity (Divine qualities).

2. *Rasatham*: It is the possession of qualities like wisdom, education, courage, justice, honesty, generosity, perseverance and austerity (Human qualities).
3. *Thamatham*: It is the possession of bad qualities like anger, laziness, lust, lying, overeating, excessive sleep, injustice, immorality, murder and stealing (Mean qualities).

Vinai—2

It means deed:

1. *Nalvinai*: Committing good deeds (*punniyam*, i.e. virtue).
2. *Thee vinai*: Committing bad deeds (*papam*, i.e. sin).

Kanma Vinai

Effects of good or bad deeds get imprinted in one's gene and are hereditarily transmitted. Depending upon the imprints, good or bad effects, or consequences occur in the successive births.

1. *Poorva Karmam* or *Kanmam*: imprints due to deeds committed in the previous birth.
2. *Sanjitha Karmam*: imprints that follow hereditarily; it accounts for the successive cycles of birth and death.
3. *Praraptha Karmam*: additional imprints due to good or bad deeds accounting for a particular birth.
4. *Kanma Noi*: example, rheumatoid arthritis, psoriasis, cancer.

The same is interpreted virtually as 'the deeds committed by parents reach (affect) their own children'. Good deeds committed in a birth produce good effects hereditarily, whereas bad ones produce bad effects or results in the successive generations.

Ragam—8
Ashta ragam means eight kinds of bad qualities:

1. *Kamam*: Excessive desire, lust
2. *Krodham*: Hatred, dispute
3. *Lopam*: Avarice
4. *Moham*: Sensuality
5. *Matham*: Madness
6. *Macharyam*: Jealousy
7. *Idumbai*: Pride
8. *Ahankaram*: Egotism

The above qualities cause diseases of the mind, body and the soul.

Avaththai—5

The five stations or positions of the soul:

1. *Nanavu (Sakkiram)*: Wakeful state
2. *Kanavu (Soppanam)*: Dreamy state
3. *Urakkam (Suzhuthi)*: Sleepy state
4. *Perurakkam (Thuriyam)*: Deep, meditative state
5. *Uyirppadakkam (Thuriyatheetham)*: *Samadhi* state (communicating with God)

Ezhu Udarkattugal—7

These are the physical constituents:

1. *Saram* (essence of digested foodstuff)
2. *Senneer* (blood)
3. *Oon* (flesh) (muscle)
4. *Kozhuppu* (fat)
5. *Enbu* (bone)
6. *Moolai* (marrow/nervous tissue)
7. *Sukkilam/Suronitham* (male/female reproductive tissue)

Panchabutham—Arusuvai—Mukkutram

(5 ELEMENTS—6 TASTES—3 HUMOURS)

Relationship between *panchabutham* and *arusuvai*

1. *Mann* (earth) + *Neer* (water) = *Inippu* (sweetness)
2. *Mann* (earth) + *Thee* (fire) = *Pulippu* (sourness)
3. *Mann* (earth) + *Vali* (air) = *Thuvarppu* (astringency)
4. *Neer* (water) + *Thee* (fire) = *Uvarppu* (saltiness)
5. *Vali* (air) + *Thee* (fire) = *Kaarppu* (pungency)
6. *Vali* (air) + *Veli* (space) = *Kaippu* (bitterness)

RELATIONSHIP BETWEEN *PANCHABUTHAM* AND *MUKKUTRAM*

Vali + *Veli* = *Vaatham*
Thee = *Pitham*
Mann + *Neer* = *Kabam*

Siddha principle says, '*Unave Marundhu Marundhe Unavu*', i.e. food itself is medicine and medicine itself is food.

There are three humours: *vali, azhal* and *iyam* (*vatham, pitham* and *kabam*). Thiruvalluvar says, *Miginum kuraiyinum noi seyyum noolor Vali muthala venniya moondru*, i.e. disease is caused either by an increase or decrease of humours. As both *suvai* and *mukkutram* are constituted by the *panchabuthams*, the imbalance of humours can be corrected by taking the foods and drugs of a specific taste.

Vali, the first humour. Its natural qualities are:

1. Producing urge or encouragement, impulse
2. Breathing in and out
3. Rendering the body, mind and speech functional
4. Exerting a driving force for expulsion or expression of 14 natural urges like defecation
5. Supporting or coordinating the functions of the seven physical constituents—*saaram, senneer, oon,* etc.
6. Giving strength to the five sense organs

N.B.: functions described under *dasa vayus*

Azhal, the second humour. Its qualities are:

It supports the body in rendering digestion, appetite, thirst, body heat, vision, taste, light (body luster), thought, knowledge, strength and softness. There are 5 types of *azhals*:

1. *Aakkanal* (*Anal Pitham* or fire of digestion): helps in the process of digestion.
2. *Vanna Eri* (*Ranjaka Pitham*): increases blood volume, gives the juice (essence) which is separated from the digested food, the typical red colour.
3. *Aatralangi* (*Saathaka Pitham*): characteristic of performing or executing an act. Located in the heart centre and with the help of knowledge, intellect and desire, it executes the desired function.
4. *Olloli Thee* (*Praasakam*): located on the skin, it gives lustre to it.
5. *Nokkazhal* (*Alosakam*): enables the eyes to perceive objects and appreciate their shape.

Iyam, the third humour. Its natural qualities are:

1. Gives strength and stability to body structures.
2. Maintains the structure and functions of joints.
3. Gives lubrication to organs during their movements.
4. Gives tolerance to an individual—to hunger, thirst, heat and other physical or mental sufferings.

There are 5 types of *iyams*:

1. *Ali Iyam (Avalambakam)*: Located in the lungs, supports the *Thirikasthanam* (lumbo-sacral and hip joints), function of the heart and the other 4 *kabams* (*avalambakam* means support).
2. *Neerppi Iyam (Kilethakam)*: Located in the stomach, it wets the foods with fluids and renders them soft.
3. *Suvaikaan Iyam (Bothakam)*: Located in the tongue, it perceives the sense of taste of foods and liquids.
4. *Niraivu Iyam (Tharpakam)*: Located in the head, it cools the eyes.
5. *Ondri Iyam (Santhikam)*: Located in the joints, it gives them lubrication and helps in extension, flexion and rotation.

In addition, there are 14 natural urges called *pathinangu vegangal*:

1. *Vaatham (Vayu* or flatulence)
2. *Thummal* (Sneeze reflex)
3. *Siruneer* (Micturition reflex)
4. *Malam* (Defecation reflex)
5. *Pasi* (Hunger)
6. *Thaaham* (Thirst)
7. *Kottaavi* (Yawning)
8. *Nithirai* (Sleep)
9. *Irumal* (Cough reflex)
10. *Ilaippu* (Hyperventilation/Exertional dyspnea)
11. *Svaasam* (Respiration)
12. *Vaanthi* (Vomiting)
13. *Vizhi Neer* or *Kanneer* (Shedding tears, crying)
14. *Sukkilam* (Ejaculation)

These urges are part of the physiological functions of the body. Their suppression will lead to morbid conditions.

Siddha also has views on embryology. These, as per *Agathiyar Vaithiya Vallathi* (verses 79–84) are: Copulation within first 14 to 16 days of menstruation, excepting the first 3 days, will result in conception. When the sperm and ovum unite, 3 *kutrams* (*doshams—vali, azhal* and *iyam*) enter the zygote as per *Dhanvanthiri Naadi* (verse 2).

The different stages of development after conception are described here:

Day 1 of gestation: Size of a mustard
Day 2: Size of a coriander seed
Day 3: Size of a pepper
Day 4: Size of a bean

Day 5: Size of a water bubble

Day 6: Size of an Indian gooseberry

Day 7: Size of a *Punnaikkai* (*Mangifera indica*)

Day 8: Formation of *panchabutham, panchavarnam* (5 colours)

Day 9: Size of a crow's egg

Day 15: Size of a hen's egg

Month 1: Size of a banana flower

Month 2: Formation of head, neck, back, shoulders

Month 3: Formation of hip, limbs, fingers and toes

Month 4: Formation of mouth, tongue and nose

Month 5: Formation of ear

Month 6: Formation of vaginal, urethral and anal orifices, nails

Month 7: 72,000 nerves and vessels, lungs, intestines, umbilicus

Month 8: Hair, supply of essence of digested food from mother to fetus, excreta through umbilical cord.

Month 9: Full life, knowledge (*Thavamuru Nilai*—worshipping form)

Month 10: Baby turns upside down (vertex presentation) and due to *abanavayu*, it is born.

Sex Determination

Regarding the choice of sex, Thirumanthiram said, *Aan migil Aanaam Pen migil pennam Poonirandothu porunthil aliyagum*, i.e. if during copulation, the affinity or love of man towards female is more, then male baby is born or vice versa; if equal, then third gender or transgender (*aravani*).

Also, if, during copulation, the breathing is along *surya kalai*, male baby will be born; if along *chandra kalai*, female baby will be conceived as per *dhanvanthiri naadi* or 18 Siddhar *naadi*.

Determination of Lifetime

As per Thirumanthiram, if *saram* flows forward from *mann* (earth) through other 4 *boothams*, the lifetime will be 100 years. If it flows forward from *neer* (water) through other 3 *boothams*, it will be 80 years. Change of flow of *saram* through each *kalai* will take place every 2 hours—on Monday, Wednesday and Friday, breathing will commence through *idakalai* from 4 a.m. On Tuesday, Saturday and Sunday, breathing will commence through *pinkalai* from 4 a.m. On Thursdays, during the spell of the waxing moon, breathing commences through *idakalai* from 4 a.m. and during waning moon, breathing commences through *pinkalai* from 4 a.m.

The flow of *saram* covers (nourishes) all the 5 elements.

ON PURITY OF MIND

Manamathu semmaiyanal manthiram jebikka vendam
Manamathu semmaiyanal vasiyai nirutha vendam
Manamathu semmaiyanal vayuvai uyartha vendam
Manamathu semmaiyanal manthiram semmaiyame

—Thirumoolar

It means that if the mind is pure, there is no need for chanting *mantras*, doing *pranayamam* or raising the *kundali*.

ON IMPERMANENCE OF LIFE

Adappanni vaithaar adisilai undar
Madakkodiyarodu manthanam kondar
Idappakkame irai nonthadhu endrar
Kidakkappaduthar kidanthozhinthare

—Thirumanthiram

This verse indicates the impermanence of life. Thirumoolar describes a so-called 'heart attack' as follows: 'A person after taking his delicious meals was chatting casually with his wife. Suddenly, indicating to his wife that he felt pain in the left side of his chest, he lay down on his bed and died at once.'

ON DEATH AND BIRTH

Uranguvathu polum sakkadu urangi
Vizhippathu polum pirappu.

—Thiruvalluvar

Thiruvalluvar, the divine poet, says, 'Death is like sleeping and birth is like waking up from sleep.'

From infancy to old age, man nurtures his body by the 96 *thathuvas* (principles) and combination of *panchabutthas* (five elements). Finally, he disintegrates into the five *buthas* from which he evolved. This incident or event is called death.

The human body, consisting of the five elements, is mortal. But the soul which leaves the body at the time of death, is immortal. Depending upon its imprints, it takes up another life.

Siddha physiology (*Udal Thathuvam*) clearly explains the nature or qualities of the body and the mind, and their relationship in health and harmony. Human birth is the rarest of all forms of births. It is only in the human birth that one can purify the soul which is attainable through purification of the mind by following ethical principles. It is only by spiritual elevation that one can maintain a harmonious relationship between the body and the mind—a healthy mind in a healthy body. Such a healthy long life leads one to self-realization and then realization of God, leading to eternal bliss, i.e. salvation.

References

Ramaswamy, R.S., *Glimpses of Thathuvam: 96 (A Handbook of Basic Siddha Principles)*.

Shanmugavelu, M., *Noi Nadal Noi Mudal Nadal Thirattu*, pts. I and II; repr., Chennai: Department of Indian Medicine and Homoeopathy, 2006.

Thiagarajan, R., Siddha Maruthuvam—Sirappu, Chennai: Department of Indian Medicine and Homoeopathy, 3rd edn., 2008.

Uthamarayan, K.S., *Siddha Maruthuvanga Churukkam*, Tamil Nadu: Siddha Science Development Committee, Government of Tamil Nadu, 2nd edn., 1983.

Venugopal, P.M., *Udal Thathuvam*, Chennai: Department of Indian Medicine and Homoeopathy, 3rd edn., 1993.

5

Thai Traditional Medicine

CHARAS SUWANWELA

THAI TRADITIONAL MEDICINE can be traced back to thirteenth century when a stone pillar belonging to the time of King Ramkamhaeng of Sukhothai was engraved with a statement concerning the use of massages for treating illnesses.

Thai medicine system was derived from both Indian and Chinese systems, and during the past 800 years, its practitioners have added their own experiences to it. The system had many gurus who wrote about it and concentrated on its practical applications and explanations.

Two systems of medicine can be recognized in Thailand. The first is the court or official system and the second is the provincial or folk system. The former can be seen from fine writing on palm leaves which were later reprinted as books called *Kampir*. More than twenty-five major books are available now, practically covering all illnesses. Some describe basic principles, anatomy and physiology, while others deal with health, longevity and causes of illnesses. There are also books which cover specific areas such as midwifery, children's illnesses, diseases of women, wind, those of the eye and even medical ethics. There are detailed descriptions covering symptoms, diagnosis, prognosis and treatment.

This folk system of medicine has many handwritten booklets. The Institute for Promotion of Thai Traditional Medicine in Thailand is launching a nationwide project to collect these writings. For instance, at the Institute of Southern Studies in Songkhla province, more than 250 writings have been collected and are under study.

Royal Backing

A major development in Thai medical system took place in 1790 when King Rama I established Bangkok as the new capital after the devastating destruction of Ayuthaya, the old one. He built Wat Po or the Wat Phra Chetuphon School of Medicine next to the Grand Palace to train new doctors. Knowledgeable people were summoned to recollect medical knowledge and figurines were made to depict it. For example, clay figures illustrating postural exercise or *rishi dad ton* were displayed on the temple ground for everyone to emulate. During King Rama III's reign in 1832, these clay figures were replaced by those made of tin and zinc alloy which exist even today.

Besides *rishi dad ton*, there were also plaques of marble engraved with herbal formulas and their uses. A building was also made which had many drawings on its walls illustrating 'lines' or meridians and their relation to health and illnesses.

However, Thai traditional medicine declined with the acceptance of Western medicine and the establishment of modern medical schools about a century back. But since 1960, the Wat Po School of Traditional Medicine has been revived and many schools of traditional medicine have sprung up. Many universities created faculties of traditional medicine and old books, illustrations and art forms on this system were revised and reinterpreted.

There are often common as well as conflicting interpretations of the Thai system and its various components since terms and wordings often have different meanings.

Elemental Stuff

According to *Kampir Thatuvipank* and *Kampir Rokanithan* which deal with basic concepts, a human being is built on four *thatu* or elements. These interact with each other like four quarter pies of a round disc which is called *chagra*. At the centre of the *chagra* is the soul. The disc rotates at a speed which is dependent on the individual's temper and changes with time and circumstances. For instance, anger makes the rotation faster. The balance of *thatu* on the *chagra* is responsible for health and harmony in life.

These *thatu* are earth (*pathavi-thatu*) which has 20 components, water (*apo-thatu*) which has 12, wind (*vayo-thatu*) which has 6 and fire (*techo-thatu*) which has 4 components. So in total, there are 42 components which make up a human being.

The earth element has 18 solid organs; water element has liquid parts of the body and includes blood, tear, nasal discharge, saliva, phlegm, sweat, urine, bile, joint fluid, thick fat, thin fat and pus. The fire element has internal fire which keeps the body warm and disappears after death, leaving a cold body. There is also external fire that allows the body to react to changing environments, fire for digestion of food and fire that burns on the body in the process of aging.

The most interesting element, though, is wind with its 6 parts— breathing in and out, wind in the belly, wind outside the bowel, wind that flows from toes up to the head, and vice versa, and wind that flows throughout the body. Wind is the force that is physically detectable. After all, breathing and bowel movement can be perceived.

According to *Kampir Tatiyapatsannibat*, there are 3 *pigat* (range or domains) of wind. First, there is *hatai-vata* or wind that keeps the body healthy and in balance. Second, there is *satathaga-vata* which is said to be the force of the mind that dictates the functioning of body *pigat*. The word *satathaga* or *shastra* means weapons. It can be a domain for defence or protection of the body. Another interpretation is a sharp change in the body like being pierced by weapons. Lastly, there is *sumana-vata*, which literally means the good mind and is the central force that pushes other *vata* to control all organs and functions. Mind and body are thus integrated as a whole existence.

What the Books Say

Kampir Samuthanvinichai deals with the causes of diseases and describes four main ones:

First is *thatu chao-ruen*, the basic *thatu* (element) governing each individual which makes one different from the other. Some *thatu* in that particular individual may be strong, while others may be weak. This can be estimated based upon the time and date of birth, which is called birth *rasi*, akin to a horoscope. The balance in each person is thus dictated at birth and can be prone to changes depending on various illnesses. Second is *ayu samuthan* where the *thatu* changes with age from childhood, middle age to old age. Therefore, it means that diseases affecting patients at different ages are different. The third is *rudu samuthan*. In this case, the *thatu* changes according to the seasons and, therefore, the diseases too are different. The fourth is *gala samuthan* where the *thatu* changes according to the time of the day.

Thatu and *chagra* imbalances lead to illnesses. One or many *thatus* can become too strong, too weak or perverted, rendering the person sick. Too strong a fire can manifest itself as fever. However, if the fire is too weak, it can affect indigestion, leading to constipation, cold and sweaty skin. Similarly, if there is turbulence in the wind element, it can cause diseases. Too strong a wind can appear as dyspnea, diarrhoea, vomiting, irritation, angry and violent behaviour and, twitching and convulsion in extreme cases. Too weak a wind shows up as constipation, difficulty in urination, mental incompetency, slow reaction, depression and paralysis.

At Wat Po, there are many pictures showing lines. They have words on the side indicative of the type of treatment used for different illnesses. A study compared these lines with meridians in Chinese medicine, and found many similarities with acupuncture points.

There are ten main lines running over the surface of the human body. These are significant to health and can be used to explain symptoms and give treatments. They start around the umbilicus and each main line has branches. Intersections of these lines are the critical points. Some say that meditation and training can lead to induction of forces along certain lines.

Lines of Importance

Line 1, *idha-chandhagala*, is on the left side. It begins below the umbilicus, goes down the front of the left leg to the tip of the toes, and then goes up along the back side of the leg to the spine, to the top of the head and then, downwards to the left nostril. It is linked to the soft gentle light of the moon.

Line 2, *pinklasuriyagala*, is similar to line 1, but is on the right side of the body. It is linked to the strong, powerful light of the sun. Line 3, *sumana*, runs from just above the umbilicus, directly upwards to the middle of the chest and neck, to end at the tip of the tongue. It is one of the most influential lines, linking the heart to the mind, as well as to speech and taste. Symptoms from illnesses pertaining to this line include mental confusion, disorientation, sleeplessness, stressfulness, speechlessness and breathlessness.

Line 10, *sukhumang kisha khigsini*, runs from the umbilicus down to the pubis and to the tip of the sex organs. This line is linked to line 3 which goes up to the tongue.

Based on these lines, massage treatments have been designed and these include caressing, percussion, pressing, and squeezing specific points. Massage treatments have also been modified with the use of herbs and aroma. The emphasis is on the surroundings and concentration on healing, by both masseurs and patients, is emphasized.

According to the Thai medical system, the mind is an integral part of the human being. Mind and body together lead to health and harmony. Mind or *sumana* flows like wind throughout the body and is the supreme *pigat* or domain. It is involved in diseases, modifies symptoms and leads to better diagnosis. The mind also plays an important part in prognosis and treatment of illnesses. Quiescence and concentration, as well as meditation, are essential for postural exercise and massage therapy.

Meditation, or manipulation of the mind, can be used to control pain and suffering from illnesses. It can also control disease processes and effect progression and outcomes of illnesses.

Glossary

Kampir: Books (example, *Kampir Tatiyapatsannibat, Kampir Samuthanvinichai*)
Rishi dad ton: Postural exercise
Thatu: Elements; there are four in the body
Chakra: A round disc, at the centre of which is the soul
Pathavi-thatu: Earth element
Apo-thatu: Water element
Vayo-thatu: Wind element
Techo-thatu: Fire element
Pigat: Range/domain
Idha-chandhagala: Line 1 (part of 10 main health lines running over the body)
Pinklasuriyagala: Line 2
Sumana: Line 3
Sukhumang kisha khigsini: Line 10

References

Bud, Book Collection of the Institute for Southern Thai Studies, Thaksin University, Songkhla, Thailand.
History of Thai Medicine, accessible at <http://www.samunpri.com/?p+17886>.
Kampir Samuthanvinichai (Causes of Illnesses), accessible at <http://www.samunpri.com/?p+17892>.
Kampir Prathomchinta (Mother and child health), accessible at <http://www.samunpri.com/?p+17995>.
Kampir Thatuvivorn (Disorders of elements), accessible at <http://www.prueksaveda.com/_m/index.pht>.
Knowledge regarding 'Kasai' (degeneration), accessible at <http://www.dtam.moph.go.th/images/document/article-panthai/kasai.pd>.
Knowledge regarding 'Thatu Chao Ruen' (the elements), accessible at <http://www.dtam.moph.go.th/images/document/article-panthai/element>.
Taosungneun, V., 'The massage therapy', *Traditional Massage,* Bangkok, 2012, p. 311.

Tengtrisom, C. et al., 'Buddhist Participating the Way to Alleviate Suffering', *Journal of Thai Traditional and Alternative Medicine*, vol. 1, June–September issue, 2003.

Thai Herbal Medicine, accessible at <http://www.samunpri.com/?cat-8194>.

Traditional Thai Medicine Textbook, 1st section, Foundation for the Promotion of Thai Traditional Medicine, College of Ayuravej Medicine, 2011, accessible at <http://www.chulabook.com/description.esp?barcode=9789748878827>.

Wiwatchankit, V., 'Diabetes Mellitus in Thai Medical Aspect', Masters thesis, Mahidol University, Thailand, 1996.

6

Buddhism and Psychotherapy

G.D. SUMANAPALA

HEALTH, BOTH PHYSICAL and mental, has become a crucial issue today. For over 2,000 years, Buddhism, Ayurveda and local traditions of medicine in Sri Lanka have rendered great service in preventing illnesses and promoting health. Together with indigenous medical systems, Buddhism plays an important role even today in promoting mental health in Sri Lanka. This article will explain the psychophysical analysis of human personality and elucidate ways of promoting health by using Buddhist and medical systems prevailing in the island. The following two definitions in Buddhism and Ayurveda will serve as the basis for preventive and promotive aspects of health.

> Ārogyaparamā lābhā—physical well-being
> Santuṭṭhi paramaṁ dhanaā—mental well-being
> Vissāsaparamā ñāti—social well-being
> Nibbāṇaparamaṁ sukhaṁ—spiritual well-being[1]

> Samadoṣasamāganiśca
> Samadhātumalakriyāḥ
> Prasannātmendriyamanāḥ
> Svastha ityabhidhīyate[2]

A healthy person is one in whom the humours, the digestive system, the seven tissue elements, waste products, sense faculties, mind and a pleasant state of soul are in balance.

The teachings of Buddha, originally delivered to people in India in the sixth century BC, have been further analysed and interpreted over a long period of time in many countries such as Sri Lanka, Burma, Thailand, China, Korea and Japan. Its purpose is to provide people with the right understanding which would be beneficial for their well being in the present life, in the life hereafter and for final freedom.

Buddhist traditions, though they vary in interpretations, commonly accept that the mental aspect of a human personality plays an important role in human behaviour. According to Buddhist analysis of the five grasping groups (pañca-upādānakkhandha),[3] mentality is explained under four groups and physical aspect under one group.

The Abhidhammic analyses the consciousness of these five groups into 89 types in one way and 121 types in another, and gives 52 psychic functions to the mentality, in relation to feelings, perceptions, dispositions and consciousness. The physical or material aspect is divided into 14 parts in early Buddhism and its Abhidhammic interpretation into 28.

The problem in this context is the term 'motivation'. The meaning or usage of the term is equivalent to the Pali term *palambhana* which means, deceiving. It means a wrong action. In the event of Nanda, the Buddha does not deceive him for any personal benefit or gain. The Pali term that applies to the situation is *samuttejana,* i.e. to gladden or to fill with enthusiasm. The term 'motivation' involves some kind of personal gain according to modern usage. Therefore, it cannot be used in the Buddhist context in order to convey the real meaning of the term *samuttejana.*

However, though mental and physical aspects are analysed as two separate groups for the sake of easy understanding, they are mutually interdependent.[4] This interdependence of the psychophysical function of the human personality, in relation to the external world, is explained in early Buddhist discourses as follows:

Step I

Physical body—External material world
Eye—Colour and shapes
Ear—Sounds
Nose—Smell (consciousness)
Tongue—Taste (mental awareness)
Skin—Temperature

Step II

Senses—sense objects—consciousness—feelings or sensations

Step III

Feelings—perceptions or memory

Step IV

Perceptions (memories)—reflection—dispositions (concepts, ideas, beliefs, views, opinions)

Step V

Senses
Sense objects
Feelings   Personality views
Perception   (Consciousness)
Reflection   (self, I-ness, soul)
Dispositions

It should be stated here that the term 'consciousness' occurs two times in the above process. It stands for the Pali term viññāṇa. The term viññāṇa in discourses does not refer to one and the same thing. In Step I, it refers to initial mental awareness as a response to contact with external objects. In Step V, the term refers to the self-view that people construct in their day to day life. Without confirmation of this view, we cannot survive in this ever-changing world. Momentary change of the psychophysical world motivates people to establish themselves permanently in the world by means of building up a personality view out of their experiences. This is the reason for their continued existence in the world in terms of birth and death. A complete stop to this process is called Final Freedom or Liberation in Buddhism.

The same psychophysical process is given a wider context in Theravada Abhidhamma and is as follows:

Step I: Stream consciousness; vibrations are formed due to the contact between senses and sense-objects and the breaking of stream consciousness.

Step II: Mental awareness arising out of particular thoughts regarding objects in relation to one of the sense faculties.

Step III: Reflection on the sense-objects in terms of accepting, investigating and determining the nature of objects.

Step IV: Mental experience or enjoyment of the sense-objects in terms of rapid succession of seven thought-moments.

Step V: Registration of the sense-experience in terms of two thought-moments.[5]

The above mentioned Abhidhammic analysis of psychophysical process includes 17 thought-moments. The complete process does not occur with regard to all experiences of sense-faculties. The moments of thought-process may vary in accordance with the extent of experiences. The mind also, as a sense-faculty, contacts mental objects or ideas directly.[6]

This mental process is different from the above to a certain extent. But this mind-door process is very important as far as the Buddhist psycho-therapeutic methods are concerned. Ven. Nyanatiloka explains the process as follows: 'The process of the inner or mind consciousness, i.e. without participation of the five physical senses is as follows: mind-object enters the mind-door (*manodvārāvajjana*), the "Impulsive Stage" and the "Registering Stage", before finally sinking into the subconscious stream.'[7]

A large number of mental problems in modern society are caused by thinking or reflecting over the concepts created through the sense data. The concepts created through the sense-perception process can be identified as mentality, mental concomitants or thoughts which are explained in the Abhidhamma as 52 *cetasikās*. Out of these, the karmically unwholesome *cetasikās* become the psychological basis for many mental problems. The 52 *cetasikās* are analysed under the following categories:

1. Karmically wholesome or neutral—25
2. Karmically unwholesome—14
3. Karmically neutral—13

Unwholesome thoughts are mainly related to greed, hatred and delusion. They become the basis for innumerable mental illnesses. Wholesome thoughts together with relevant behaviour provide a good ground to get rid of all such problems.

According to early Buddhist teachings, human beings possess two mental tendencies by birth—likes and dislikes. These are mental reactions and they are extremely useful and essential for the survival of beings. Further, they are not harmful defilements. But, problems arise when they are developed without limits. The unlimited growth of these two aspects is shown in Table 6.1

TABLE 6.1: Unlimited Growth of Likes and Dislikes

Normal level	Middle level	Final level
likes	greed	covetousness (discontent)
dislikes*	hate	malevolence (desire to injure)

Note: *Ven. Nyanatiloka, *Buddhist Dictionary*, Singapore, 1946. See under *Cetasika*.

Middle-level tendencies are considered as mental disorders or unwholesome mental roots and final tendencies are treated as unwholesome mental functions.[8] As a result of unlimited development of greed and discontent, one wishes to get everything one likes. Due to the changing nature of the world, no one is able to get everything they wish. As a result of this failure, delusion arises in the mind. On the other hand, due to the development of hate and malevolence, this attempt also becomes unsuccessful due to the impermanent nature of the world, though one wishes to keep away everything that one does not like.[9] The result is same as in the first case. So, delusion or mental disorder (confusion) becomes a common factor of all unenlightened beings. Hence, the Buddhist saying that all ordinary beings are like mad people.[10]

Together with this madness, there arises another defilement called conceit.[11] Delusion and conceit are basic factors of mental disorders. All mental problems, whether they belong to psychosis or neurosis, can be explained in relation to these mental reactions. In brief, this is the basis of psychotherapy in Buddhism.

Therapeutic Methods

There are some specific characteristics that serve as the basis for therapeutic methods in Buddhism.[12]

1. All psychotherapeutic methods in Buddhism are directed towards nibbāna—extinction of all defilements. The actual experience of the goal is to give up everything in order to end the suffering caused by repeated existence or rebirth. The patient who holds this view is able to bear any problem with patience and satisfaction because he is not trying to gain anything but trying to give up everything.

2. Even a single mental illness is not named in Buddhism. Instead, the basic or root elements of mentality are explained mainly with reference to the above mentioned unwholesome and wholesome roots. All mental problems depend on these basic elements. There are three main reasons for not naming mental illnesses:

   • Physical illnesses are durable and they can be easily identified, while mental illnesses are momentary and cannot be identified with certainty.
   • It is the nature of human beings that they depend on concepts indicated by specific terms to confirm their existence. Once they attach words such as stress, depression or phobia to a mental

BUDDHISM AND PSYCHOTHERAPY 59

illness, the same word becomes as though the mental illness itself. Mental illness is thus identified by some characteristics, it never exists permanently. Searching for characteristics to identify a certain mental illness is an unsuccessful attempt. But the problem is that without naming an illness, one cannot prescribe a medicine. For Buddhism, the mind is a specific faculty in the human personality and is not only related to the brain but to all five physical sense faculties.

- Buddhist psychotherapeutic methods are mainly directed at changing the mentality of persons. They do not pay much attention to changing the environment or other external or physical factors in order to calm the mentality.

Three Stages of Psychotherapy

The practice of psychotherapy is also based on a simple formula which can be expanded and extended to any mental problem. The practice has three gradual stages:

1. Development of moral behaviour—behavioural therapy
2. Development of concentration—psychological therapy
3. Development of understanding—cognitive therapy

The first type of therapy refers to restraining of the five senses which are mainly responsible for physical and verbal behaviour of man.[13] The second type refers to restraining of mental disorders, namely greed, hatred and delusion-conceit.[14] The third type of therapy concerns the development of understanding in people regarding the true nature of the world of experience.[15] These three stages are mutually interconnected and support restraining and development of each aspect gradually. Therefore, in Buddhist practice, these three stages should be connected with every method of psychotherapy.[16]

It is not out of context to mention the relationship of the physical body with the above three stages—greed, hatred and delusion. The *Bhesajjamañjusā*, the only Pali Ayurvedic work available, states that mental health should be maintained in accordance with the *Tripiṭaka*. *Bhesajjamañjusā* instructs to establish physical health. According to Ayurveda, all physical illnesses are related to imbalance of the three humours—phlegm (water), bile (yellow bile-fire; black bile-earth) and blood (air). The *Visuddhimagga* mentions that these three are connected with mentality as:

- Greed—leads to phlegm
- Hatred—bile
- Delusion—blood[17]

Although there are many other causes and conditions that influence physical health, such as environment and food, mental condition plays a prominent role in balancing the physical condition.

It is a fact that any theory cannot be put into practice as it is. So Buddhist psychologists can devise and develop various methods to be used in Buddhist psychiatry. All of them should be in conformity with the basic elements of Buddhist theory and practice of psychotherapy. Though all such methods bring temporary effects, complete recovery of all mental problems can be achieved only through the realization of *nibbāna*, the *summum bonum* of Buddhist path to freedom.

Until the final realization, we should use such methods and I have developed some depending on Buddhist cultural accounts. These methods are taught in postgraduate courses in our University of Kelaniya and have been used in Sri Lanka in counselling programmes for over three years.

1. *Confession*: This method is derived from the practice of *āpattidesanā* is followed by Buddhist monks and nuns. If they commit anything wrong, they have to declare it in front of another member of the Saṅgha society before the dawn of the next day. Accumulating the experiences of wrong actions create mental problems. So it is better to purify one's mind by declaring every such incident and making this a daily practice.

2. *Imitation*: Iavaka and Aṅgulimāla—these two well-known characters in Buddhist canon were tamed by Buddha first by agreeing with them. (Iavaka saw Buddha sitting in his cave and ordered him to go out.) Buddha followed his order three times and finally he was converted to Buddhism. According to this method, we should agree with the behaviour of the mental patient, otherwise we cannot control the patient as we wish.

3. *Generalization*: Some people think mental problems only affect them. They become calm when they understand that such problems are common to many. Kisāgotamī, who was mad about the death of her son, realized the common nature of death when she was asked by Buddha to bring some mustard seeds from a house where no one had died.

4. *Kamma* (*law of nature*): This Buddhist theory is a good therapeutic method that can be adopted successfully. There are

some mental problems that cannot be analysed properly as they do not reveal all causes and conditions. In such cases, we may explain that Kammas related to former lives, may influence the present life. After experiencing the effects of such Kammas, we will be released from such effects in future. This way of thinking has created a contented society for over 2,000 years in Buddhist countries.

5. *Dialogue*: In many discourses of the canon such as Kasiûbhāradvāja and Aggañña, there are friendly, logical and philosophical dialogues of Buddha with various people. These dialogues have helped eliminate mental problems in different types of people.

6. *Noble silence*: In some cases, the best method of treatment is to maintain complete silence without responding to the complaints made by patients. This has solved many social and individual problems in Buddhist society.

7. *Psychoanalysis*: With reference to Madhupiṇḍika, Mahānidāna sutta, etc., the counsellor should analyse the psychological process of the patient in order to clarify the causes and conditions of the problem.

8. *Right motivation*: According to the famous event of Nanda, he was taken to heaven by Buddha in order to detach him from Janapadakalyāṇi by showing damsels. The theory behind this method is that one cannot totally detach from a concept at once. So the person should be motivated to achieve a higher goal and from there, he should be directed to the desired object.

9. *Logical analysis*: Some educated people like to argue with others. So the method of argument can be adapted to eliminate their problems. Āseṭṭhasutta and Aggañña sutta are good examples in this regard.

10. *Innocent punishment*: Brahmadaṇḍa is a punishment in which all other members do not talk to the patient. This can be used mainly for those with personality disorders such as anger and arrogance. The main feature of these punishments is that they never hurt the patient physically.

11. *Praising*: Some people suffer due to lack of appreciation for their work. They should be directed to a suitable environment where they are appreciated. Before passing away, Buddha did not forget to appreciate Ven. Ananda's service and the benefits of the last meal given by Cundakammāraputta.

12. *Friendly meeting*: Some people suffer mentally due to lack of association with other people. They should be provided friendly meetings with suitable persons.

13. *Creating religious emotions*: Pilgrimages are one of the most suitable ways of creating religious emotions in order to get rid of mental problems such as worry, guilty-conscience, sorrow, etc.

14. *Creating emotion and intellect*: This concept is called *Vedalla*. Here, the patient is provided with occasions where he can experience happiness and knowledge in tandem. Reading novels, watching drama, singing, dancing, etc., can be used.

However, the application of all these methods should be in conformity with the threefold therapeutic measures—behavioural therapy, psychological therapy and cognitive therapy. These measures are termed the middle path.[18] It avoids the two extreme ways of living, i.e. self-mortification and self-indulgence.[19]

Aṣṭāṅgahṛdaya, a famous Ayurvedic text, recommends the middle path in every human action as a healthy way of living.[20] The middle path is also explained as the noble eightfold path.[21] These include: cognitive aspects, right view, right thoughts, behavioural aspect, right speech, right action, right livelihood, psychological aspect, right effort, right mindfulness[22] and right concentration.

The practice of the behavioural aspects of the above path is recommended in *Aṣṭāṅgahṛdaya* and is as follows: refrain from killing, stealing, sexual misconduct, tale-bearing, harsh words, lying, useless talk, ill-will, greed and wrong view.[23]

Both the Buddhist path and Ayurveda emphasize the importance of ethical behaviour for promoting health, as well as for preventing the causes of illness. Further, almost all Ayurvedic texts written in Sri Lanka and India devote some chapters for ethical codes as an essential part for the establishment of a healthy society.

The other two therapeutic ways, namely, psychological therapy and cognitive therapy, are applied with the specific purpose of promoting mental health, though they are also beneficial for maintaining physical health.

Abbreviations

A—Aṅguttaranikāya
D—Dīghanikāya
M—Majjhimanikāya
MA—Majjhimanikāya Aṭṭhakathā
S—Saṁyuttanikāya

Notes

Except indicated otherwise, all references refer to the editions of the Pali Text Society, London.

1. *Dhammapada*, ed. and tr. Ven. K. Dhammananda, Taiwan, 1988, p. 405.
2. Three humours: phlegm, bile and air.

   Seven tissue elements:

   rasa—chyle including lymph
   rakta—the haemoglobin fraction of the blood
   māṁsa—muscle tissue
   medas—fat tissue
   asthi—bone tissue
   majjā—bone marrow
   śukra—the sperm in male and ovum in female
   From Vaidya Bhagawan Dash, *Fundamentals of Ayurvedic Medicine*, Delhi, 1978, p. 28.
3. S. 111., p. 101; D. 111., p. 233; M. 1., p. 190; A.V., p. 52.
4. G.D. Sumanapala, *Abhidhammic Interpretations of Early Buddhist Teachings*, Singapore, 2005, pp. 12–14.
5. G.D. Sumanapala, *Early Buddhist Philosophy and Social Concepts*, Singapore, 2001, pp. 8–11.
6. G.D. Sumanapala, *An Introduction to Theravāda Abhidhamma*, Singapore, 1998, 135–7.
7. Ven. Nyanatiloka, *Buddhist Dictionary*, Singapore, 1946. See under Viññāṇakicca.
8. Anunaya, paṭigha, D. 111., p. 254; M. 1., p. 191; D. 1., p. 25; A. 1., pp. 3, 87, 200.
9. Akusalamūla, Akusalakamma.
10. *Ummattako viya hi puthujjano*, MA. 1., ed. Hevawitharana, Colombo, p. 23.
11. Māna, D. 111., p. 234.
12. *Adhivacanasamphassa*, D. 11., p. 62; M. 1., p. 113; D. 111., p. 86.
13. Sīla, D. 111., p. 235.
14. Samādhi, A. 111., p. 12.
15. Paññā, D. 1., p. 245.
16. S. 111., p. 83.
17. *Visuddhimagga*, ed. Ven. Saddhatissa, Colombo, 1914, p. 76.
18. *Vinaya*, i, Pali Text Society, London, pp. 10–11.
19. Ibid.
20. *Aṣṭāṅgahṛdaya*, tr. Ven. P. Pemananda, Colombo, 1939, p. 21.
21. Vinaya, i, Pali Text Society, London, p. 11.
22. *Path of Purification*, tr. Bhikkhu Nanamoli, Taiwan, 1956, p. 582.
23. *Aṣṭāṅgahṛdaya*, Pemananda, p. 19.

7

Diagnosis and Imbalances in Traditional Tibetan Medicine

NAMDOL LHAMO

With Compassion, serves all sentient beings,
'O Enlightened One' mere hearing your name,
Relieves the sufferings of all lowly births;
Healer of the diseases of the three inborn mental poisons,
To the enlightened supreme healer,
'The king of Aquamarine Light' I prostrate before you.

—'Words of Homage to the Medicine Buddha' in *Gyueshi*

TIBETAN MEDICINE IS a rich traditional medical system, which is more than 2,500 years old. It evolved from its own culture, diet, lifestyle habits, religion, environment and resources. Later, it also integrated essences from medical traditions of neighbouring countries such as India, Persia and China, thus making it one of the most comprehensive and well synthesized medical system.

Tibetan medical system has a close relationship with the outer macrocosm and inner microcosm as both evolved from the same material basis of five elements. The two greatly influence each other in various aspects, such as issues related to the ecological state and the well-being of living beings. Besides, the diseases that humans suffer from, and their remedies and therapeutic methods are also based on the same fundamental five elements. Therefore, human beings, diseases and remedies share a common principal basis.

Synthesis of Body and Mind

In this medical system, a human being forms from the union of sperm and ovum, and consciousness. These collectively make an amalgam of the body and mind—one of the indications to claim that psychology is already incorporated in Tibetan medicine since its origin. The relationship between body and mind can be compared to that of a supporter and its dependent, or a house and its inhabitant. Both are highly dependent on each other for their well-being and act as a controlling force, throughout the lifespan.

The human body is physiologically made up of three principal energies (*nyepa sum*), and ten bodily components (*noeja chu*). The three principal energies are *loong* (wind), *tripa* (bile) and *baekan* (phlegm). The ten bodily components comprise of seven bodily constituents (nutritional essence, blood, muscles, fats, bones, marrow, and regenerative fluid), and three waste products (faeces, urine and sweat). Their fundamental bases are the five elements (earth, water, fire, air and space) and mental consciousness has its perpetual continuum from that of its previous lives.

When these energies and bodily components are present in balanced quantities and coordinated functions, it results in a balanced state of health. However, if the opposite happens due to the adoption of an unwholesome diet and lifestyle, it results in diseases or imbalances.

Diagnosis, an indispensable part of health care, can be done through three main techniques:

1. Diagnosis based on aetiological factors

Generally, there are four main causative factors which trigger diseases. They are diet, lifestyle, season and evil spirits. However, certain diets and lifestyles are the specific causes of disorders. It is based on the law of cause and effect.

2. Diagnosis based on the signs and symptoms of a disorder

The relationship between a disorder and its signs and symptoms is like that between fire and smoke. Just like fire can be identified by smoke, a disorder can be identified by its own signs and symptoms. Any physician who is ignorant of diagnostic techniques will not understand the signs of a disorder and its true manifestations. It is similar to smoke being mistaken for steam or falsely predicting rain whenever clouds gather in the sky. Consequently, uncertain signs could be taken for real ones, resulting in wrong diagnosis.

3. Diagnosis based on assessing the effects of the given treatment

This is based on prolonged assessment of the effects of treatments given in the form of diet, lifestyle management, medicines and external therapies.

Expert Diagnosis

There are three main diagnostic methods:

1. Visual examination

This examination is made through all the objects seen by the physician with his naked eye. This includes the patient's body structure, height, appearance, complexion, physical and mental expression, characteristic signs of the sensory organs and their functions, and characteristic signs of sputum, stool, vomit, blood, tongue and urine.

The tongue can reveal a lot too. In the case of *loong* disorders, the tongue is generally red, dry and coarse, with small pimples. In *tripa* disorders, the tongue is covered with thick and pale yellowish coating and in *baekan* disorders, it is pale, moist, and smooth, with a thick whitish coating and excessive saliva.

Urine analysis, too, reflects the state of health and is explained in eight sections: preliminary instructions on diet and lifestyle activities; the appropriate time for urine examination; qualities of a required urine container; process of urine transformation; healthy urine; unhealthy urine; urine indicating impending death and urine indicating evil spirit influences.

A urine sample is basically checked for its colour, vapour, smell and bubbles when it is freshly warm. When lukewarm, it is checked for sediments (*ku ya*) and scum (*tri ma*) and when cold, for time, process and characteristics of transformation. Generally, urine is clear like water with big bubbles in *loong* disorders, reddish yellow, with strong vapour and smell, and thin bubbles, which disappear quickly in *tripa* disorders, and whitish with minimal smell and vapour, and lasting saliva like bubbles in *baekan* disorders. Urine examination is specifically known to help determine whether the disorder is of a cold or hot nature because of the sediment constituent in it, which is the metabolic byproduct of blood and bile.

2. Examination through touch

It includes examining the temperature, growth and texture of body parts, and pulse analysis. Pulse is like a messenger between the physician and the disorder, and its analysis is explained in thirteen sections: preliminary instructions on diet and lifestyle activities; appropriate time for pulse examination; proper place for finger placement; pressure of the fingers to be applied on the pulse; methods of pulse examination; three constitutional pulses in healthy persons; four seasonal pulses in relation to the five elements; the seven pulses in healthy persons; examination of healthy and unhealthy conditions based on the number of pulse beats; identification of general and specific pulses; pulse indicating an impending death; pulse influenced by evil spirits and examination of lifespan through life force (*laa*) pulse.

Usually, the radial artery on the lateral side of the wrist is examined for diagnosis, whereas the ulnar artery on the medial side of the wrist is palpated for examining the state of one's life force or lifespan. The dorsalis pedis artery on the dorsal part of a foot is used for diagnosing an impending death. Pulse analysis is known to accurately predict life or death. Generally, the pulse in *loong* disorders is floating and empty with halting beats, thin, fast and twisted in *tripa* disorders, and sunken and slow with declining beats in *baekan* disorders.

3. Examination through interrogation or history-taking

It includes questioning—which, how, where, what, when—of causes and conditions, locations of diseases, and signs and symptoms of a disorder. This is because causes and conditions help to diagnose a specific principle energy which is deranged in a disorder. Locations of diseases help to determine the pathway of a disorder, and signs and symptoms help to verify the specific disorder.

So, in order to obtain appropriate therapeutic results and to cure the patient, we must prepare him properly for diagnostic procedures. Traditional Tibetan medical system has rich and sophisticated diagnostic methods such as pulse and urine analysis, besides emphasizing the great importance of history, during all the processes of disease investigation. As our fundamental medical text *Gyueshi* says, 'For all the various diagnostic methods, history-taking through interrogation is highly mandatory and important.' Thus, for a physician, history taking equips him with the tricks and skills to diagnose any disease through knowing the causes of a disorder, signs and symptoms of a disorder, and from the histories of diagnosis made, as well as treatments taken in the past.

To conclude, I would say that diagnosis in Tibetan medicine is very comprehensive and covers all the diagnostic possibilities which can be implemented in not only the treatment of the disorders, but also for their prevention.

References

Clark, Barry, *The Quintessence Tantras of Tibetan Medicine*, USA: Snow Lion Publication, 1995.

Clifford, Terry, *Tibetan Buddhist Medicine and Psychiatry—The Diamond Healing*, New Delhi: Motilal Banarsidass Publishers Pvt. Ltd., 1994.

Clinical Research Department, Men-Tsee-Khang, *Tibetan Medical Dietary Book*, Dharamshala: Men-Tsee-Khang, vol. I, 2006.

Dawa, *A Clear Mirror of Tibetan Medicinal Plants*, Dharamshala: Men-Tsee-Khang, vol. I, 1999; vol. II, 2009.

Dekhang, Tsering Dorjee, *A Handbook of Tibetan Medicinal Plant*, Dharamshala: Men-Tsee-Khang, 2008.

Donden, Yeshi, *The Ambrosia Heart Tantra*, tr. Jhampa Kelsang (Alan Wallace), Dharamshala: Library of Tibetan Works and Archives, 1977.

———, 'Pulse Diagnosis in Tibetan Medicine', *Tibetan Medicine*, no. 1 (translated from the first chapter of the fourth Tantra), Dharamshala: Library of Tibetan Works and Archives, 1980, pp. 13–29.

———, *Health Through Balance*, Ithaca: Snow Lion Publications, 1986.

Drungtso, T. Thakchoe, *Basic Concepts of Tibetan Medicine—A Guide to Understanding Tibetan Medical Science*, Dharamshala: Drungtso Publication, 2007.

Fundamentals of Tibetan Medicine, Dharamshala: Men-Tsee-Khang, 4th edn., 2001.

Norbu, Namkhai, *On Birth and Life: A Treatise on Tibetan Medicine*, English tr. Dr Barry Simmons, Italy: Tipografia Commerciale Venezia, 1983.

Parfionovitch, Yuri et al., *Tibetan Medical Paintings*, New York: Serindia Publications, 1992.

Rabgay, Lobsang, 'Pulse Analysis in Tibetan Medicine', *Tibetan Medicine*, no. 3, Dharamshala: Library of Tibetan Works and Archives, 1981, pp. 45–52.

———, 'Urine Analysis in Tibetan Medicine', *Tibetan Medicine*, no. 3, Dharamshala: Library of Tibetan Works and Archives, 1981, pp. 53–60.

Translation Department, Men-Tsee-Khang, *The Root Tantra and the Explanatory Tantra of Tibetan Medicine*, Dharamshala: Men-Tsee-Khang, 1st and 2nd edns., 2011.

8

Naturopathy and Yoga

Diagnosis and Imbalances

B.T. CHIDANANDA MURTHY

HEALTH AND HEALING have taken complicated overtones today. It is because of the increasing number of diseases, countless drugs and their combinations, different systems of medicines, new investigations, diseases being detected at an advanced stage and growing specialization. In addition, there is the increasing burden of health on a population where 70 per cent still cannot access medical facilities and many clearly lack medical insurance. Will we then ever reach an optimal level of health as seen in countries abroad?

Though we have made a breakthrough in emergency medicines, particularly for accident cases, many acute and chronic diseases are still a challenge. So much so that we see longevity without any quality of life. In this context, it is evident that the basic approach to health systems needs to be revised. Understanding the basic philosophy of health and healing is, therefore, essential.

All cures are brought by nature. Many species have lived for centuries with the aid of self-curative powers and this is the philosophy of nature cure or Naturopathy and Yoga. It is simple, safe, has long-term benefits and is curative.

According to the WHO, 'Health is not merely the absence of disease or infirmity, but a feeling of well-being at the physical, mental, social and spiritual levels.'

The philosophy of nature cure is based on natural laws and principles which are also normally followed by all animals and birds and have their applications in life, death, health, disease and cure.

Principles of Nature

According to the principles of Naturopathy, violation of nature's laws results in lowered vitality, accumulation of morbid matter and abnormal composition of blood and lymph. Naturopathy, therefore, is the readjustment of the human body from abnormal to normal conditions by detoxification. The accumulation of foreign matter which is unwanted manifests itself as disease, while its elimination leads to cure.

The human body is the product of five elements and should live in accordance to the principles of Mother Nature. In case this is violated, we are bound to be sick. To regain health once again, we should take the help of these five elements:

1. Earth—Exemplified by tissues, muscles and bones and comprise about 30 per cent of the body.
2. Water—Body fluids, blood, lymph, which comprise about 65 per cent.
3. Air—Oxygen and carbon dioxide.
4. Sun—Body temperature, gastric juices.
5. Ether (cavities)—Lungs, stomach, intestines, uterus, urinary bladder.
6. Universal Soul.

Each of these elements has a corresponding nature cure. The help of air is taken with fasting and air bath; water (hydrotherapy), ether (fasting therapy), earth (mud and diet therapy), and fire (sun and colour therapy).

Naturopathy is a wonderful, drugless therapy based on sound scientific principles. According to it, the body has remarkable, recuperative and regenerative powers and if scope is given, it can heal itself as it has self-healing forces.

From various researches, it is evident that drugs are more dangerous than diseases. Besides, they are costly, give temporary relief, create iatrogenic diseases (caused by abuse of drugs and doctors), suppress the disease and lead to inertia in healing oneself. Patients take health for granted and think they can purchase it. In fact, 90 per cent of diseases are due to faulty eating habits and can be brought under control by proper diet. These habits lead to toxins getting accumulated in the body.

Three-Dimensional Science

Naturopathy is a holistic science which has a three-dimensional approach—preventive, curative and rehabilitative. Hence, it is very important for its practitioners to have faith, positive thinking, willpower, patience and perseverance. The role of a Naturopath is to aid the healing process through natural remedies only. Many scientific researches are being carried out in the West where diet, hydro, mud and massage therapy have had beneficial effects on various diseases.

Mahatma Gandhi was a great believer and advocate of nature cure. He said, 'Nature Cure has been a passion with me since childhood. To serve the cause of nature cure has been the dream of my life ever since. Around 999 cases out of 1,000 can be brought round by a mean of regulated diet, water, air, sun and earth-treatments and similar household remedies.'[1]

Naturopathy promotes natural, organically grown, and fresh food items. We all are aware of the hazards of pesticides, food colours, highly refined and deodorized (non-nutritious) food which are also carcinogenic. In this scenario, awareness and demand for natural food will bring a revolution of good food habits and lead to its availability.

Nature cure has three stages:

1. *Eliminative stage*: Includes enema, hip bath, *pranayama*, walking, *asanas* and fasting therapy.
2. *Soothening stage*: Fruitarian, vegetarian diet, hydriatic applications (baths, massage, steam bath).
3. *Rejuvenative/constructive stage*: Individual-tailored dietetics, Yoga, baths, etc.

Naturopathic diagnosis is based on taking the full case history, facial diagnosis, iris diagnosis (which will indicate the condition of various visceral organs), modern clinical diagnosis and chromo diagnosis (changes in the colour of skin, eyes, urine, faecal matter).

Eyes and Health

Iridology is the examination of colours and other characteristics of the iris to determine a patient's health. Genetic strengths and weaknesses, levels of inflammation and toxicity, and efficiency of organs all build a picture of current health status and predispositions.

Practitioners match their observations to iris charts, where zones correspond to specific parts of the human body. Iridologists see the eyes as windows into the body's state of health. They believe they can use the charts to distinguish between healthy systems and organs and those that are overactive, inflamed or distressed. This information demonstrates a patient's susceptibility to certain illnesses, reflects past medical problems and predicts future ones.

The iris, incidentally, is the greenish-yellow area surrounding the transparent pupil (the black area in the eye). The white outer area is the sclera and the central transparent part, the cornea. Iridologists generally use flashlights, magnifying glass, cameras and slit-lamp microscopes to examine a patient's irises for tissue changes as well as look for specific pigment patterns and irregular stromal architecture.

Typical iris charts divide it into approximately 80 to 90 zones. For example, the zone corresponding to the kidney is in the lower part of the iris, just before the 6 o'clock position seen in a clock. There are minor variations in charts between body parts and areas of the iris.

According to iridologists, details in the iris reflect changes in the tissues of the corresponding body organs. One prominent practitioner, Bernard Jensen, said, 'Nerve fibers in the iris respond to changes in body tissues by manifesting a reflex physiology that corresponds to specific tissue changes and locations'.[2] This would mean that a bodily condition translates into a noticeable change in the appearance of the iris. For example, acute and chronic inflammatory and catarrhal signs may indicate involvement of corresponding tissues.

Worldwide Phenomenon

The first use of the word *augendiagnostik* ('eye diagnosis' is loosely translated as Iridology) began with Ignaz von Peczely, a nineteenth-century Hungarian physician. In fact, Iridology began in Hungary. Peczely got the idea for this diagnostic tool after seeing similar streaks in the eyes of a man he was treating for a broken leg and in the eyes of an owl whose leg he had broken many years before.

The Germans too had a contribution to make here. Pastor Emanuel Felke, a minister, had developed a form of homoeopathy for treating specific illnesses and described new iris signs in the early 1900s. Pastor Felke was subjected to a long and bitter litigation. The Felke Institute in Gerlingen, Germany, was established as a leading centre of Iridological research and training.

Iridology became better known in the United States in the 1950s when Bernard Jensen, an American chiropractor (trained health professional who uses a variety of non-surgical treatments), began giving classes in his own method. This was done along with P. Johannes Thiel, Eduard Lahn (who became an American under the name of Edward Lane) and J. Haskell Kritzer. Jensen emphasized the importance of the body's exposure to toxins and the use of natural foods as detoxifiers.

Medical research in several European countries and Russia, in particular, have established greater acceptance of Iridology. In Russia, a trial involving 8,00,000 patients found Iridology to be 85 per cent accurate in diagnosis. In South Korea, clinical trials by the government found that on an average, Iridology was 78.20 per cent accurate, but with an impressive 90.20 per cent accuracy in the diagnosis of digestive disorders. By contrast, orthodox medicine considers other diagnostic techniques as reliable if they are accurate within a range of 30–40 per cent.[3]

The iris and pupil are one of the most complex structures in nature and also some of the most visible. They have thousands of nerve endings which are connected to the brain through the hypothalamus, enabling one to determine conditions in all organs and systems of the body. The iris provides accurate information about our constitution. When bodily tissues become inflamed or congested, the iris is able to register the processes, enabling the iridologist to determine the root cause of the disorder. For example, a toxic digestive system may be responsible for problems such as migraines, skin disorders or joint problems. In India, research is essential so that this diagnostic system can be popularized.

Read the Face

Facial Diagnosis is another diagnostic method used in Naturopathy. It is the ability to determine the physical status of a person from external appearances. It can help discover the location and amount of foreign matter in the body. Louis Kuhne, a German Naturopath, says, 'The science of facial expression concerns itself with the whole organism. There is no disease affecting only a particular part of the body. In every illness, the entire system suffers. The whole body changes in form and colour, but this alteration is only sufficiently pronounced for clear observation at certain places.'[4]

Kuhne observed old Greek sculptures which were beautiful as human forms and from them, he derived notions of health and ill-health. The following theory was established from these observations: a healthy man's body and mind should function properly without pain and without artificial stimulations or drugs. These functions, necessary for maintaining life, include absorption of food and expulsion of waste material. The healthy man experiences a feeling of hunger, which is satisfied by the consumption of natural foods. This feeling of satisfaction occurs before there is any uncomfortable sensation of fullness and the process of digestion goes on quietly just like those of absorption and elimination. There is sound sleep and on waking up, the person is cheerful, bright and content.

The normal figure of a healthy person is proportionate. The head is of moderate size and the neck is round, neither too short nor too long. No prominences will be noticed on it and its circumference will be roughly equal to that of the calf of the leg. The chest is arched, the abdomen is not prominent nor is the trunk prolonged downwardly. The legs are strongly built and bowed neither inwardly nor outwardly. The forehead is free of wrinkles, is smooth and has no adipose cushion. The eyes are clear and free from veins.

In judging the body, mobility is also important. There should be natural, unhindered movement. The head should be capable of free left and right movement. There must be no tension at the nape of the neck when it is lowered.

However, foreign matter in the body shows itself through different encumbrances and has led to the Encumbrance Theory. There are four types of encumbrances:

1. Front Encumbrance
2. Side Encumbrance
3. Back Encumbrance
4. Mixed Encumbrance/Whole body encumbrance

Signs in Body Shapes

Front encumbrance concerns itself mainly with the front portions of the body. The neck is usually too full in front and the face, enlarged and clumsy. Sometimes it is only the mouth that protrudes, the foreign matter having settled there alone.

The facial boundary is the jawline, sharply defining the face from the neck. In a normal person, it runs directly from the chin, outlining the jaw, up to the ear. In cases of front encumbrance, this natural boundary line is either pushed back or is more or less obliterated. The deviation from the normal is in direct proportion to the degree of encumbrance. If front encumbrance predominates, the face looks bloated and a fatty cushion may form on the forehead.

The encumbrance of the forehead plainly indicates that the foreign matter has reached the region of the brain. In some cases, lumps have developed upon the neck, though these may, in time, reduce in size, and the emancipation of the muscles may restore the jawline to its normal distinctness.

There are other such definite lines observed in a normal body, namely, one that separates the back of the head from the neck, and another between the thigh and abdomen. In a normal, healthy person, the skin can be easily raised from the forehead. There is nothing between it and the bone. But in a case of encumbrance, a layer of fat seems to be inserted, and it is almost impossible to move the skin. The formation of small, raised pimples often follow. The condition of the forehead is sometimes the result of back encumbrance, when the foreign matter has risen along the spine, and crossed the top of the head, settling in the upper portions of the face. When the front encumbrance exists, the complexion is either pale or unduly red. The parts most encumbered show great tension and a shiny appearance. In this condition, there are diseases of the neck, throat, lungs, eyes, head, etc.

In the case of side encumbrance, there is a distinct enlargement of the neck on the side which is affected. Often all the parts on that side are broader, so that the whole body appears asymmetrical. If the foreign matter is accumulated in the right side of the body, the entire right side of the face is larger than the left. This is noticeable in the legs as well, and, consequently, the line of the head is not in the centre of the body. The affected leg is not sharply defined from the body, and considerable enlargement is found on the thigh line. By degrees, the head will grow perceptibly one-sided, and lumps will probably form on both sides of the neck. The encumbered side is indicated by tension in the muscles, produced by turning the head from one side to the other. Not infrequently, vertical cords or strings appear in the neck, indicating the course of the foreign matter. The consequences of side encumbrance are more serious and more difficult to cope with as it affects the spinal cord, and symptoms include severe headaches, and eye and skin problems.

In the case of left-sided encumbrance, rheumatism and gout will generally be there. This is especially so, if aggravated by back encumbrance as well. In that case, the kidneys which act as depurating (cleansing) organs of liquid effluvia, will become affected and fail to purge the system. The heart also suffers in left-sided encumbrance, especially when coupled with frontal encumbrance.

Back encumbrance too has various symptoms. The head is too large and bent forwards. The forehead is cushioned, the eyes protrude and the nose is normal. The chin and mouth are too thick, the jawline is absent and the nape line is missing. The back is a sort of cushion and round-shouldered so that it looks like a hump.

Back encumbrance is usually accompanied by piles and as the hips are afflicted, the gait is staggering. This encumbrance has acute symptoms and the patient's only hope is in profuse perspiration and immediate and energetic use of eliminating baths. As soon as back encumbrance reaches the region of the head, nervousness, lack of attention, loss of memory and lack of energy are manifested. These people are usually very active and restless in the early stages. They are often hypochondriacs, and considered as specimens of ill-health on account of their bloated body and flushed complexion. Problems related to infertility, menstrual cycle and impotence occur with back encumbrance. Disorders of the spine become chronic and the gait of the person becomes slow and the body protrudes forward.

In the case of mixed and universal encumbrance, front and side encumbrances are found together. Side encumbrance may be connected with encumbrance of the back. Front and back encumbrance may be present in the same individual. Of course, the afflictions of those suffering from universal encumbrance are more serious. These people are nervous, restless, discontented, and predisposed to acute ailments. They might die suddenly, though, on account of their appearance of stoutness (owing to the presence of so much foreign matter), they are usually thought to be in excellent health. In treating them, chances of recovery and rapidity of cure depend a good deal upon age and general vitality. The bloated condition of the body renders treatment more effectual.

In universal encumbrance, the head is too large and the forehead, cushioned. The eyes are normal, the nose is too thin, the mouth is a little open and the jawline is absent. The neck is enlarged all around and immovable. The nape line is obliterated. There will be considerable swelling behind the ear. The shoulders will be sloping to a high degree. Diseases associated with this encumbrance are digestive disorders such as constipation, IBS (irritable bowel syndrome), ulcers, colitis, acidity, etc. There will be malabsorption and general disability. Problems related to joints are also prominent.

All the encumbrances indicate the type of diseases, duration, severity and number of days required to detox the body. Treatment is started in three phases: Eliminative, Soothening and Constructive. In each phase, depending on the condition of the encumbrance, treatment is provided. Modalities tried include fasting, natural dietetics, hydrotherapy, mud therapy, sun and colour therapy, acupressure, acupuncture, exercise therapy, massage, physiotherapy and Yoga. Fasting has been found to have many benefits in bringing down the encumbrances.

In conclusion, nature is often the best teacher.

Notes

1. Mohandas Karamchand Gandhi, *The Story of My Experiments with Truth*, Navajivan Publishing House, 1990, p. 226.
2. Bernard Jensen, 'Iridology Simplified', 2nd edn., Escondido California: Whitman Publications, 1980, p. 3.
3. A Report from Complementary Health Care Information Service, UK, www.highimpact.my/public/apps/page/index.php? id=S1-1631 4212.
4. Louis Kuhne, *Handbook of the Science of Facial Expression or the New System of Diagnosis*, translated from the German edition, Leipsic: Louis Kuhne, 1902, p. 20.

References

Jensen, Bernard, *The Science & Practice of Iridology.*
Kuhne, Louis, *The Science of Facial Expression.*
———, *Neo-Naturopathy.*
Lindlahr, Henry, *Iridiagnosis & Other Diagnostics.*
———, *Philosophy of Nature Cure.*
———, *Practice of Nature Cure.*

9

Homoeopathy

Diagnosis and Imbalances

MOHAMMAD QASIM

ANCIENT INDIAN PHYSICIAN Charaka said, 'A physician who fails to enter the body with the lamp of knowledge and understanding can never treat diseases.' Later, in the early eighteenth century, the father of homoeopathy, Dr C.S.F. Hahnemann said, 'The physician's high and only mission is to restore the sick to health, to cure. . . .'[1]

Healing, therefore, is a task which cannot be taken lightly. The human body is a paradox of which we know little, though it always comes up with astonishing surprises. The science of the human body is intricate; it is healthy in functioning, with smooth and coordinated performance of the mind. It has creative energy and can be a source of pleasure to the eye of an artist.

However, with the onslaught of disease, the body and mind end up in a state of turmoil. Both states, health and sickness, are manifestations of the body as a whole unit. The body, through its functions, gives various signals about where and why things have gone wrong. In *The Principles and Art of Cure by Homoeopathy*, Dr Herbert A. Roberts writes:

The whole body is sick, not a cell of an organ, but the organ as a whole. Homoeopathy embraces the cause of the diseased condition, the course of the condition and its prognosis. The method of approach is based upon the knowledge of the patient, the knowledge of the remedy and comprehension of the laws of health and disease. Homoeopathic concept of the disease and cure . . . considers the broad outlines of the whole rather than some of the minute divisions comprised by the whole.[2]

Individualized Treatment

Intelligent people realize the prize of individuality and those who have struck out on their own hold better opportunity to help the suffering. Homoeopathy, in this regard, offers an individualized method of treatment in chronic illnesses. The disease is largely due to a deficit in the immune system, thereby making the person vulnerable to outside or inside invading agents. As the body becomes defenceless, building up the immune system becomes a long process. In due course, it is strengthened and fortified.

Thus, homoeopathy provides hope for many illnesses that are long-standing and seemingly incurable. Building the immune system is possible simply by the mode of preparation of medicines, special knowledge of their application and recognizing the diseases and their mode of development. Diagnosis is threefold:

1. Diagnosis of the disease—Pathological
2. Diagnosis of the patient—Clinical origin of the disease
3. Diagnosis of the remedy—Matching the patient

Medical science is the art of listening. Just being heard by the physician reduces half the discomfort of the patient. This valuable art is lost due to technical advancement. Giving a patient hearing to the sick person is part of therapy. After all, the symptoms are due to some turmoil inside the body which will be articulated by the patient. The methodology of treatment depends on how the symptoms are presented. Past illness, family history and the emotional quotient of the patient help an observant physician in analyses of the illness. The condition of the disease can alter according to the emotional stress and strain of the patient.

Homoeopathy is deeply in touch with the spirit of nature and nature of the human spirit because human beings are part of nature and respond to changes in the environment.

Cardinal Principles

Certain cardinal principles must be followed while taking down the history of the patient. The first principle is location, sensation, modalities, and concomitant. Location means the place where the disease is located, sensation indicates the quality of pain, modalities provide the time of occurrence or aggravation of the pain, discomfort or fever and concomitant means any other sign or symptom not related to the chief features of the disease. These four essential points make the diagnosis. In a recent case of cold and cough, the patient said that he had been plagued by these symptoms all the time and no physician had been able to cure it. 'Can you help me resolve the uneasy feeling in the chest? I feel as if my heart is hanging from a thread', he said.[3] While these seem to be odd symptoms, they are often encountered in homoeopathy practice and there is no explanation for them. There are other similar symptoms which physicians often ignore. All these have specific roles in diagnosis and the selection of final remedy.

The second principle is finding out how susceptible one is. Homoeopathic physician explores the nature of the person as a whole—the emotional and physical sensitivity and susceptibility. This has a direct relation to the circumstances and environment he has been brought up in and those in which he is presently living. The influence of these factors can be evaluated in the origin of the disease. For example, if peeling an onion causes running of the nose, sneezing, watery eyes and flushed face, then the patient is susceptible and sensitive to onions. Interestingly, susceptibility and sensitivity are archaic words, and these have been modified to allergy.

Allergy is an exaggerated reaction to a thing to which there is no reaction normally. Homoeopathic medicines play a pivotal role in controlling this exaggerated reaction. Susceptibility and sensitivity can be emotional as well as physical, and can be manifested as IBS (irritable bowel syndrome), ulcerative colitis, increased heartbeat, high blood pressure, skin, respiratory distress, etc. The physician has to then take on the role of investigator and dig deep into the emotions of the patient in order to heal him.

Extent of Exposure

The intensity of symptoms varies from person to person depending on the quantity and time of exposure. While some may react to the exposure for a short duration, others may take time to show symptoms. This explains the predisposition of the patient to react in a given situation. This is an idiosyncrasy manifested any time with any substance, taken either internally or exposed externally. Idiosyncrasy is an explosive condition of the constitution wherein the individual reacts strongly to different harmless substances. This reactive power of the person is used to observe the toxic effect of the medicinal substance and can be applied to similar clinical conditions of the person.

In homoeopathy, it is more important to identify the cause of not feeling well emotionally than to know the agents causing allergy. A depressed mind makes the body easily susceptible to illness. On the other hand, the reactive power of the patient's immune system as well as the homoeopathic medicine together act promptly, smoothly and harmlessly. Homoeopathy, therefore, makes the mind and body stronger so that it can resist foreign invasion. It changes the character of thinking and body behaviour.

Minute doses of the medicine with higher dilution are more suitable in reaching the mind and touching the emotional plane of the patient. This, in turn, helps to restore health. The medicine acts through nerve ends which carry the memory of the vitalized medicine to the brain and then to the affected area. Through the nerves and blood vessels, the medicine reaches difficult zones of the human system and brings an effective change in the thinking process of the patient, to ultimately heal him.

The fourth principle is classification of the disease. This is crucial for curing. This theory is unique in the management and treatment of illnesses. Dr Hahnemann evaluated and experienced it before putting it to test. In my practice over forty years, this theory has been closely verified by patients.

Past History

The knowledge of whether diseases such as psora, syphilis, sycosis, tuberculosis and cancer have been predominant in the past or in the family gives leverage in the management of sickness. This is the single most advantage that this science has in dealing with all kinds of difficult and incurable cases. This makes it relatively easy to reach a possible cause for the illness, no matter what its name. The name of the disease is only an identity of the condition, but not the means of treatment.

Similarly, selection of medicine keeping in mind the past history of the patient and family illness in cases such as glioma (a type of brain tumour), epilepsy, multiple sclerosis, gastric disorder, migraine, etc., has brought a new lease of life to the sick. For example, in cases of brain tumour, it is important to trace the period of health and sickness of the patient to give a clue about the line of treatment to be taken. Illnesses suffered before the actual tumour manifested itself are important and the extent of recovery can be a guiding force in assessing the present condition. Based on this analysis, carefully selected remedies for the present condition have yielded good results.

If nothing is found in the patient's past illness, then the family history should give a clue. Habits, lifestyle, emotional strain, sleep patterns and digestive and respiratory susceptibilities give evidence of the predominant disease or the likely weaknesses in certain areas of the body that may cause it. Invariably, I have found diseases in the family of a patient which have helped me relate the disease to appropriate areas in the body.

A disease of chronic nature has its root in an acute condition which can be temporarily alleviated. Nonetheless, the acuteness remains dormant in some form. To illustrate this point, there was a case of a fifteen year old patient with brain tumour. She had developed this after she was treated with a full course of anti-tubercular drug. Her mother had suffered from tuberculosis of the lung and been give full ATT (anti-tubercular treatment). The girl was treated along these lines with homoeopathic medicines and subsequent MRI of the brain showed improvement. Finally, the growth was healed. This relationship between diseases and past family history has been found in many chronic cases.

Division of Diseases

The division of various diseases has been adopted from the classification of different things in nature, be it animals, plants or minerals. For all chronic diseases, the following categories have been formulated:

1. *Psora*: A condition which has its roots in skin disorder.
2. *Syphilis*: A venereal disease characterized by a variety of lesions in which the chancre (sore) and mucous patch are distinctive. Its favourite seats are over the flat bone, membranes of the brain, liver, spleen and testis. Another less important lesion produced by syphilis is diffuse sclerosis of the blood vessels. In some remote cases, there is cutaneous eruption, sore throat, general enlargement of the lymph nodes and a systemic toxemia (all these are differing expressions of one root cause). There are some secondary manifestations which may be lesions in the form of aneurysm of the aorta, interstitial keratitis (corneal scarring due to inflammation) and involvement of the central nervous system which manifests itself as meningitis, tabis dorsalis (degeneration of the nerves), etc. In some cases, though no active syphilitic lesion was seen, syphilitic eye (ulceration) was noticed by eye specialists and homoeopathic prescription has yielded good results. Syphilis is further confirmed when the patient shows a history of urogenital disease in the past. Anti-syphilitic medicine is then given and the eye saved.
3. *Sycosis*: An inflammatory disease affecting the hair follicles, particularly the beard and characterized by papules, pustules,

tubercles and crusting. This disease has been prevalent since ancient times due to living conditions, food habits, environmental changes and above all, personal and social living habits. These three mixed miasma (environment), psora, syphilis and sycosis, lead to more complicated manifestations such as tuberculosis and cancer.

4. *Tuberculosis*: This condition has various effects on prominent organs of the body, skin, lungs, bones, spine, nervous system and brain.

5. *Cancer*: Another version of chronic disease whose cells invade easy targets of the body. It has its roots in past illness of family members and exposure to environment. It is the result of wrong eating and living habits, causing great emotional and physical stress.

It is obvious that homoeopathy's methodological approach signals big hope to patients.

Notes

1. Samuel Hahnemann, *Aphorism 1, Organon of Medicine,* tr. R.E. Dudgeon, 5th edn., Calcutta: M. Bhattacharya & Co., p. 115.
2. Herbert A. Roberts, *The Principles and Art of Cure by Homoeopathy,* Bradford, Holsworthy, Devon, England: Health Science Press, 1942, p. 259.
3. H.C. Allen, 'Kali Carb', *Keynotes of Characteristics with Comparison of Some of the Leading Remedies of the Materia Medica*, 8th edn., Philadelphia: Boericke and Tafel, 1950, p. 154.

References

Blakiston's Illustrated Pocket Medical Dictionary, ed. Normand L. Hoerr and Arthur Osol, 2nd edn., McGraw-Hill, 1960.

Lown, Bernard, *The Lost Art of Healing: Practicing Compassion in Medicine*, Random House, 1998.

Roberts, Herbert A., *The Principles and Art of Cure by Homoeopathy*, Bradford, Holsworthy, Devon, England: Health Science Press, 1942.

10

Homoeopathy

Therapies and Treatments

ESWARA DAS

HOMOEOPATHY HAS BECOME a household name in India and a distinct medical specialty practice across the world. It has become a recognized medical system in our country through the Homoeopathy Central Council Act, 1973. Known for its safety and gentle effect, homoeopathy has blended well with the roots and traditions of the country. Its strength lies in its effectiveness in certain clinical conditions for which there is little or no other treatment. Besides, it takes a holistic approach to sickness by promoting inner balance at the mental, emotional, spiritual and physical levels.

During the last 50 years, homoeopathy has been successfully institutionalized in India. It has a highly commendable infrastructure with 185 teaching institutions, 2.2 lakh registered practitioners, 414 drug manufacturing units, an autonomous research council with 32 peripheral units, a regulatory council for quality education at the university level, drug safety regulations, laboratories, committees, and primary and secondary health care facilities.

Homoeopathy was formally propounded and systematized as a distinct new medical system by German physician Dr Christian Friedrich Samuel Hahnemann in 1796. 'Homoeopathy' comes from the Greek words *hómoios* (similar) and *páthos* (suffering), i.e. 'Similar sufferings'. It is based on the principle *similia similibus curentur*, which means 'let likes be treated by likes'. This implies that the disease-producing powers of a substance can be used to treat natural diseases which exhibit similar phenomenon.

Homoeopathy can be defined as a 'dynamic, holistic and vitalistic system of individualistic drug therapeutics, based on the law of similars, potentially capable of curing cases that are curable and relieve symptoms of incurable nature'.[1] Its crucial principles are the doctrines of drug-proving and drug-dynamization theory of chronic diseases, totality of symptoms and direction of cure. The important supporting principles are vital force or dynamism, single remedy and susceptibility or individualization.

Hahnemann, the Father of Homoeopathy

Dr Hahnemann (10 April 1755–2 July 1843), the founder of homoeopathy, was also an expert in eight languages—German, Latin, Greek, Italian, French, Spanish, English and Arabic. He was a studious medical observer. After graduating with an MD from the University of Erlangen in 1779, he practiced medicine till 1784, but became disenchanted with the imperfections of medical practice and left clinical practice.

However, he had great interest in chemistry and originated several innovations, becoming an acclaimed chemist. He used his talents in languages and chemistry to satisfy his inquisitiveness about the world, people and other cultures. This helped him open a unique window into the medical systems and traditions of other cultures. He could translate medical works of other cultures and, thus, gain wide knowledge of their drugs and uses. From 1777 to 1806, he translated twenty-four textbooks and numerous articles into German, usually accompanied with extensive footnotes and detailed corrections of his own.

In 1790, Hahnemann started translating Cullen's *Materia Medica*, where he came across the medicinal effects of Peruvian bark, whose astringent, but property had a tonic effect on the stomach. Hahnemann's curiosity made him suspect that there were stronger bitters and stronger astringents which did not have the properties of curing ague (malaria or other illnesses involving fever and shivering). Hahnemann became indignant over the theoretical explanations of the antipyretic (pertaining to fever) property of cinchona bark and experimented upon himself. He took an ounce of cinchona bark tincture and was surprised to see that the symptoms emerged were similar to marshy fever. He slowly became convinced that a substance which could cause a disease-like state could also cure a similar condition. After doing several experiments on healthy humans, patients and himself, he was convinced that a better and safer system of treatment could be offered to mankind based on natural laws.

Based on experiments, Hahnemann codified a new paradigm in medical practices in 1810 and published the *Organon of the Healing Art* wherein he laid the foundation of the theoretical and practical aspects of homoeopathy. And, thus, was homoeopathy born.

Guidelines for Homoeopaths

Hahnemann revised the *Organon* by updating his experiments and later six editions were published, of which five were during his lifetime. From the second edition onward, the name was changed to *Organon of Medicine*. It contains 294 aphorisms.

In the theory part of *Organon of Medicine*, he laid down the highest ideal of cure, the principles of mission for the physician, requisite knowledge for a homoeopathic physician and its application to disease, knowledge of remedies, modes of treatment and reasons for superiority of homoeopathic therapeutics.

In the practical part, he codified three points necessary for curing, classification of disease and case-taking. These included recording patient's data, knowledge of medicinal power, curative power, most suitable method of employing medicine to a patient, allied support during treatment, diet in acute diseases, preparation and administration of medicines and Mesmerism.

Hahnemann wrote many books. These were: *Organon of Medicine* (six editions), *Materia Medica Pura* (two volumes), *Chronic Diseases: Their Peculiar Nature and their Homoeopathic Cure* and *The Lesser Writings of Samuel Hahnemann* (a collection of his writings).

During his lifetime, many stalwarts got attracted to his new principles. They contributed to the further development of homoeopathy. Some of the early contributors were Dr John Henry Clarke, Dr James Tyler Kent, Dr Constantine Hering, Dr E.A. Farrington, Dr Charles Julius Hempel, Dr Henry C. Allen, Clemens Maria Franz Von Bönninghausen, Dr Timothy Field Allen, Cyrus Maxwell Boger, Dr J.C. Burnett, Carol Dunhum and Stuart Close.

Concepts and Principles

The law of similars: Also called the law of cure, it demonstrates that the selected remedy is able to produce a range of symptoms in a healthy person similar to that observed in a patient, thus leading to the principle of *similia similibus curentur*. The principle has been verified by millions of homoeopaths all over the world.

The concept of single remedy: This law directs to choose and administer a single remedy which is most similar to the symptoms of the sick person.

The law of minimum dose: The similar remedy selected for a sick person should be prescribed in a minimum dose, so that when administered, there are no toxic effects on the body. It only acts as a triggering and catalytic agent to stimulate and strengthen the existing defence mechanism of the body. It does not need to be repeated frequently.

Holistic as well as individualistic approach: Homoeopathy does not treat the disease per se. A homoeopath does not concentrate his therapy on say, arthritis or bronchitis or cancer, or for that matter to painful joints, inflamed bronchi or a malignant growth. Rather, a homoeopath treats all mental, emotional and physical aspects of the patient. Homoeopathy regards each patient as a unique individual. Therefore, two persons with hepatitis may get two different homoeopathic remedies, each one aimed at the individual's totality of symptoms rather than his liver alone. The physician's interest is not only to alleviate the patient's present symptoms but to look for his long-term well-being.

Concept of vital force: Hahnemann discovered that the human body is endowed with a force that reacts against inimical forces which produce disease. It becomes deranged during illness and the well-selected remedies stimulate this failing vital force so that, as Hahnemann said, 'it can again take the reins and direct the organism on the way to health'.[2]

Concept of miasm: Psora, syphilis and sycosis are the three fundamental causes of all chronic diseases and are called miasms. This word is derived from the Greek word *miainein*, which means 'to pollute'. Syphilis and sycosis are venereal and contagious chronic diseases, whereas psora is a non-venereal chronic disease. Psora persists from the beginning to the end of life and is the root cause of most diseases.

Principle of drug-proving: To apply drugs for therapeutic use, their curative powers should be known. In homoeopathy, drugs are proved on healthy humans first before being applied to patients. The symptoms thus known are the true record of the curative properties of a drug or the pathogenesis of a drug.

Drug-dynamization or Potentization: Drugs are prepared in such a way that they retain maximum medicinal powers without producing any toxic action on the body. It was found experimentally by Hahnemann that when diluted drugs are powerfully succussed (shaken), they develop lasting medicinal powers.

March of Homoeopathy

Homoeopathy gained a massive following in the United States during the late nineteenth century. In 1844, the American Institute of Homoeopathy was formed, becoming the first national medical organization there. Homoeopathy gained recognition because of its success in treating many epidemic diseases rampant at that time, including scarlet fever, typhoid, cholera and yellow fever. Statistics indicate that the death rates in homoeopathic hospitals from these epidemics were often half to as little as one-eighth when compared to those in orthodox medical hospitals.

Homoeopathy reached Asia, including Russia and the Indian subcontinent, in the early nineteenth century. In India, it gained a foothold owing to its successful use in cholera and other epidemics. Homoeopathic dispensaries, hospitals, educational institutes and pharmacies opened in all parts of India and it became the system of the common man.

This therapeutic system spread around the world almost in step with colonial powers, missionaries and travellers within a relatively short period. It had similarities of approach with prevailing traditional and ethnic medicinal systems in colonized nations and easily merged with them. The nineteenth century, thus, saw the proliferation of homoeopathic hospitals, colleges and pharmacies in many parts of the world.

In India, homoeopathy can be traced to early nineteenth century when German missionaries treated people on the shores of Bengal. The first account of treatment, however, is mentioned in the travelogue of John Martin Hongberger (physician to the Court of Lahore), titled *Thirty-five Years in the East: Adventures, Discoveries, Experiments and Historical Sketches Relating to the Punjab and Cashmere; in Connection with Medicine, Botany, Pharmacy &c*. He treated Maharaja Ranjit Singh of Punjab in 1839 with homoeopathic remedies.

Its initial success in cholera and other epidemics in Bengal made it popular among the common man. Charitable dispensaries and hospitals were opened, and private practitioners, either disciples of experienced homoeopaths or those who were self-learnt, started practising it. The system received a further impetus with the establishment of educational institutions and pharmacies.

Great Strides

The system also owes recognition to the concerted efforts of some eminent Allopathic doctors who opted for homoeopathy and used it with remarkable success. The efforts of a few institutionally trained homoeopathic physicians also paved the way for the then Bengal Provincial Government to establish the General Council and State Faculty of Homoeopathic Medicine in 1943.

Post-independence, the legislatures of Indian states began enacting laws to regulate teaching, practice and research in homoeopathy. These include the Madras Registration of Practitioners of Integrated Medical Act of 1956 and the Mysore Homoeopathic Practitioners Act of 1961. State legislatures made them responsible for strengthening colleges, hospitals, dispensaries and pharmacies dealing with Indian systems of medicine and almost all states established Directorates of Indian Medicine for the development of traditional systems. At the Centre, indigenous systems of medicine became a part of the Ministry of Health and Family Welfare and their growth was made legitimate by including them in the Five Year Plans.

The Homoeopathic Research Committee constituted in 1963 initiated the process of organized homoeopathic research and identified priority research areas. A combined council to conduct research in Indian systems of medicine and homoeopathy was formed initially in 1969. This paved the way for individual research councils and subsequently, the Central Council for Research in Homoeopathy was formed in 1978. The Council identified broad areas of research and evolved protocols over the years to develop homoeopathy in the country.

The Homoeopathy Central Council Act, 1973, established the legislative mechanism to regulate homoeopathic practice and education in India. This ensured that physicians are trained as per norms and their practice is regulated. The National Institute of Homoeopathy was established at Calcutta in 1975 as a model institute for undergraduate and postgraduate education and research. The Homoeopathic Pharmacopoeia Laboratory was also founded in 1975 to lay down principles and standards of preparation of homoeopathic drugs. Due to sustained efforts of the government, an institutional framework for homoeopathy has been established at the Centre as well as in all the states.

Solid Cure

Not many know that homoeopathy can cure many illnesses of serious natures also. There is a good amount of documentary evidence on its benefits in cancer, HIV/AIDS, chikungunya, infertility, sinusitis, asthma, allergies, etc. Documentation needs to be followed up with adequate and carefully designed clinical research which should then lay down guidelines for the management of clinical conditions. It should further disseminate strategies of management for different health conditions while respecting the basic principle of individualization.

Today, every medical discipline is facing challenges with the resurgence of resistant chains of organisms, more invasive diseases, emergence of new diseases like HIV/AIDS and an increase in lifestyle problems. Homoeopathy may be a viable option as a stand-alone treatment or as an adjunct in many of these clinical areas. Therefore, what is required is integration of homoeopathy with other healthcare modalities, improving the curriculum to meet the above objectives and reorientation of teachers of homoeopathy colleges.

What is needed in future is to explore the role of homoeopathy in epidemics. This has become a dire necessity as evidenced by the recent upsurge of the H1N1 influenza and the consequent panic because of it. Most state governments were wary of allowing access to the homoeopathic profession to examine affected patients. This is in sharp contrast to the proactive measures adopted by Kerala through the constitution of REACH (Rapid Epidemic Action Cell in Homoeopathy), which becomes active at the first sign of an emerging public health problem and is empowered to disseminate information and advise officials.

Looking at the enormity of the task, the government alone will not be able to do everything in creating a need-based health care system. The need of the hour is to search for competent organizations and individuals who can forge partnerships among themselves so that they can utilize their expertise for formulation, implementation and evaluation of the problem. Public-private partnership schemes have been formulated by the Department of AYUSH to provide an educational, clinical and communitarian base for the development of institutions. Through these schemes, research, teaching and health care delivery are promoted and several collaborative programmes are implemented in the country.

Prevention is Better than Cure

Just as the *similia* principle is the universal law for curative care, there are universal principles for prevention and promotive aspects in homoeopathy. Sociologists believe that improvement in the health status of the community is brought in through an integrated approach of various stakeholders, including the community, social organizations, voluntary health care agencies, social psychologists, etc. The paradigm advocated by sociologists is that of a community oriented health care delivery system with physicians acting as facilitators for the development of the community.

Community health is concerned with the surroundings rather than the individual. Providers of this service have to go to the community unlike in clinical medicine where the patient seeks the intervention of the physician. In individual-based health care, instant therapeutic intervention is given importance. But preventive health is more holistic and directed towards the entire population and community. It is more cost effective. A judicious preventive health system will drastically reduce the burden of diseases, especially among the poor in developing countries.

Preventive interventions are implemented through a universal concept of *Genius epidemicus* which states that the most indicated curative medicine in any case of epidemic, endemic or sporadic event will be the preventive medicine for that event during that season.

Homoeopathy gives much importance to the constitution, temperament and miasmatic background of the individual. Any dyscrasias (disease/disorder) at any of these three levels might derange the health of the individual. Adequate care to address the dyscrasia will save the individual from falling sick. Thus, constitutional or anti-miasmatic remedies are used in promoting the health of the individual.

Conclusion

Homoeopathy is a system of medicine with the potential strength to cure several diseases and encourage preventive and promotive aspects of health care on established scientific principles. The system is cost effective, gentle in its therapeutic modalities and based on the holistic concept of mind, body and spiritual framework of the sick. The system follows a unique concept of individualization of the patient and pursues the principle of totality of the symptom as the key to selecting remedies.

However, one of the major criticisms the system faces is its inability to explain certain concepts like vital force, theory of drug-dynamization, minimum dose, etc. Nonetheless, homoeopathy has withstood the onslaught of its critics for over two hundred years and established many of its concepts as valid and scientific. Efforts are going on to find plausible answers to the remaining intricate questions with the help of recent advances in science like biotechnology, nanotechnology, quantum physics, etc. Whatever be its shortfalls, the popularity of homoeopathy is increasing and the demand for its services expanding.

The future of health care delivery will be pluralistic and the system neutral, wherein every recognized medical system will contribute to its strength and the public shall avail these services in an integrative manner. In that manner, homoeopathy will continue to play an important role.

Notes

1. Definition taken from National Health Portal website, http://www.nhp.gov.in/.
2. R.E. Dudgeon, *Lectures on the Theory and Practice of Homoeopathy,* London: Aylott & Co., 1983, p. 76.

11

Tibetan Medicine

A Holistic Approach to Health

I strongly believe that our medical system is one of the means by which we Tibetans can contribute to the well-being of others, even while we ourselves live as refugees.

—His Holiness the Dalai Lama

THERE CAN BE NO statement as apt as this to describe the universal appeal of Tibetan medicine. Ever since mankind existed in this universe, it has been dependent on nature for sustenance and survival. Bereft of any knowledge of the sciences, it survived through primitive methods. First, man learnt how to light a fire and cook his food. Eventually, he developed his thinking by instinct and intuition, and discovered remedies for common ailments from local herbs. He documented this, leading finally, to many healing systems of medicine.

This knowledge was passed from generation to generation, with each system of medicine having its own diagnosis, treatment and explanation. By the late 1900s, everyone, rich or poor, realized that medicine could help improve one's quality of life, which had become stressful. Indigenous systems started evolving, using different logic and techniques of healing. But the aim was always the same—to heal and cure mental and physical illnesses.

Tibetan medical system is one of the oldest traditional forms of medical system. It has been preserved and practised for more than 2,500 years and is a major area of study in Tibet. So, it is an integral part of Tibetan life and culture and great kings, saints, scholars and physicians propagated it and laid a solid foundation for it. By extracting the essence from other traditional healing systems, an authentic Tibetan medical text *rGyud-bZhi* or the Four Tantras was complied.

Tibetan medicine is science, art and philosophy all rolled in one. It is a science because its foundation is laid down in a systematic and logical way, based on the understanding of our body and its relationship to environment. It is an art because it uses various diagnostic techniques to identify health problems and uses a therapeutic measure to maintain proper and optimal health; and it is a philosophy because it embraces key Buddhist principles such as altruism, karma and ethics.

Tibetan medicine has two theories. One is the psychical, *Dug gSum* (three mental poisons or three negative emotions) and other is cosmo-physical—*'Byung-baNga* (cosmo-physical elements). Psychical theory is related to the mind and holds that everything within the universe is in a constant state of flux. All phenomena are characterized by impermanence and their only permanent feature is impermanence. Buddha also traced the root cause of all suffering to the concept of Ignorance, which obscures our mind from understanding the Law of Causality and Reality of Phenomenon. Therefore, the first and foremost thing that we have to understand and recognize is the mind, its emotions and its nature.

Ignorance literally means the non-existence of the self. Due to this, one suffers from three inborn mental poisons—desire, hatred or anger, and delusion or confusion. This gives rise to various forms of imbalances in the body. These can be grouped under *rLung, mKhris-pa* and *Bad-kan*. Just as the bird is never separate from its own shadow, the sentient being will never be free from illness because of the presence of ignorance even though the person may be living with joy.

There are two aspects of the mind—fundamental and ordinary. The fundamental mind is luminous, indefinite, pure and clear, like a mirror. It has no form, shape and colour. Every being possesses this kind of mind and is therefore akin to Buddha. The ordinary mind, on the other hand, has no form, shape and colour because it has no solid ground. Its negative emotions are transitory and one can eradicate them by spiritual practices. Here, the fundamental, pure, and clear light of the mind is polluted by negative emotions as a result of which, different emotions afflict the ordinary mind. While the fundamental mind can be compared to a clear sky, the ordinary one is like a cloud.

Tibetan medicine is based on the concept of five elements—earth, water, fire, air and space. Earth is the basis for the origin of substances. Water has the attributes of moisture, which is present in most substances.

Fire is heat, which provides optimal temperature for ripening and maturing. Air stimulates growth and movement, while space ensures that development takes place. These five elements are also present in anatomy and physiology. Therefore, our body is composed of five cosmo-physical elements. When the body is healthy, these five elements are in equilibrium with each other. However, if there is an increase or decrease in these elements, then the body becomes imbalanced. Because of an improper diet and unwholesome lifestyle, the three humours, *rLung, mKhris-pa* and *Bad-kan*, come in turmoil and make the body unhealthy.

Even the beginning of human life, caused by the union of semen of the father and ovum of the mother, has contributions of the mind, *Kun shinamshe* (storehouse of consciousness), the imprint of the past *karma* action force of afflictive emotions and the five cosmo-physical elements. While the semen contributes to the formation of the skeletal tissue, the brain and the spinal cord, the ovum helps form muscles, tissues, blood and vital organs. One has to understand the formation of the body by elements. The earth element forms the flesh, bone, nose and sense of smell, whereas water forms blood, body fluids, the tongue and a sense of taste. Fire provides heat or temperature in the body and determines complexion and forms the eye. Air is responsible for respiration, formation of skin and a sense of touch. Finally, space forms the various channels, ear and a sense of hearing.

Mind or consciousness is a multilayered, multifocal capacity with roots in evolution. The true nature of our consciousness is as vast as the cosmos. This is what Buddhism teaches. Today, top scientists are engaging with Buddhist philosophy to investigate and research various mental stages and emotions. More and more neuroscientists are trying to investigate the nature of the mind and its mental projections, but they have a long way to go before reaching the truth.

According to Buddhism, at the gross level of consciousness, we have 84,000 emotions in our body which correspond to the functioning of the brain and interaction of the body with its environment. The gross levels of consciousness include five sensory ones: eye, ear, nose, tongue, body consciousness and mental consciousness. In our day-to-day life, we can experience different transitory feelings by using the sense faculties. For example, with eye consciousness, we can see various objects and different visuals; with nose consciousness, we get a sense of smell; with ear consciousness, a sense of hearing; with tongue consciousness, an experience of taste; with body consciousness, a sense of touch and with mental consciousness, we get different mental projections.

Tibetan medicine states that body and mind co-exist on three principal energy (three *Nyes-pa*) levels. While they support our life, when imbalanced, they cause malfunctions in the seven bodily constituents and three excretions, resulting in physical and mental suffering. In fact, twenty-five bodily aspects have to be in equilibrium for us to have a healthy mind and body. The body is connected to the channels, the channels to *rLung* (wind energy) and *rLung* to the mind. *rLung,* of which there are many, is responsible for physical and mental activities such as respiration, development of body, delivery of the foetus, menstruation, spitting, speech, sense organs and sustaining life by acting as a medium between the mind and the body. The five *rLung* reside on central nervous systems of the body and are called the main energy centres or chakras: These chakras are, crown chakra, throat chakra, heart chakra, naval chakra and genital chakra. Ultimately, if these *chakras* function properly, then the physical body is healthy, and then the channel functions remain optimum and there is proper movement of *rlung* with the channels. The mind remains alert and fresh; *rlung* energy moves smoothly within the body and enhances the functions of the channels. In return, it boosts the health of the person.

References

Donden, Yeshi, *Health through Balance*, Ithaca: Snow Lion, 1986.
Donden, Yeshi and Wallace B. Alan, *Healing from the Source*, Library of Congress Catolging-in-Publication Data, 2000.
Dummer, Tom, *Tibetan Medicine and Other Holistic Health-Care Systems*, New Delhi: Paljor Publication, 2001.
Fundamental of Tibetan Medicine, Dharamshala: Men-Tsee-Khang, 2000.
Gonpo, Yuthok Yonten Gonpo, *rGyud-bZhi* (Four Tantras), Tibet People's Press, 1992.
Gyalpo, Sukar Lodoe, *Mepoi Shellung (Comentary on rGyud bzhi)*, Dharamshala: Men-Tsee-Khang, 1992.
Gyatso, Sangyal, *Bay-nyon*, vols. I–II, Dharamshala: Men-Tsee-Khang, 1997.
Phuntsok, Thupten, *Bhoe-kis sorik-nyingnor-chaytue*, Zikhron People's Press, 1996.
Tsenam, Toru Rinpoche, *rGyud-bZhi Del-Chen (Commentary on rGyud-bZhi)*, Zikhron People's Press, 2000.
The basic Tantra and the Explanatory from the Secret Quintessential Instruction on the Eight Branches of the Ambrosia Essence Tantra, Dharamshala: Men-Tsee-Khang, Translation Department, 2008.

12

Traditional Medicine in Myanmar

Preventive and Promotive Aspects

AUNG MYINT

M YANMAR IS BLESSED with a traditional system of medicine. For over 2,000 years ago, it has flourished in many parts and has been prevalent from the earliest periods such as Tagaung, Srikestra and Bagan. The teachings of Buddha as well as traditions and customs, geographical conditions and availability of raw material from plants, minerals, animals and marine sources have led to its growing influence.

This system has a number of profound medical treatises, effective medicines and diverse therapies. The longevity of Myanmar people is a testimony to the potency of its traditional medicine.

Myanmar traditional medicine has four components. The first one is *Bhesijjanaya*, an Ayurvedic concept, which flourished in cities such as Tagaung, Srikestra and Hanlin during the early periods of Myanmar civilization. At the beginning of the Bagan Era, the Abhidhamma-based *Desananaya*, *Netkhattanaya* and *Vijjadharanaya* branches of medicine took root.

The *Desana* system is based on natural phenomenon of hot and cold. Its concept largely depends on Buddhist philosophy, with the therapeutic use of herbal and mineral compounds, and diet. The *Bhesijja* system employs extensive use of herbal and mineral compounds, to establish balance among the three *doshas*, namely, *vata, pitta* and *kapha*. The *Netkhatta* system is based on zodiac calculations of the stars, planets and the time of birth, and age. These calculations are then linked to prescribed dietary practices. The *Vijjadhara* system is largely dependent on meditation and practices of alchemy.

The skill, know-how and techniques of drug preparations are derived from heavy metals, such as lead and mercury, and poisonous substances (arsenic and its compounds). These are converted into inert ones by means of chemical processes in order to obtain supernatural power.

The Beginning

In 1953, an office to promote traditional medicine was established under the Department of Health and finally, in 1989, a separate Department of Traditional Medicine was established under the Ministry of Health. The objectives of the department were:

1. To provide the entire nation with comprehensive traditional medicine services through the existing health care system in line with the National Health Plan.
2. To develop a standardized method of therapeutic criteria systematically.
3. To review and find out ways and means for newly developed therapeutic agents and medicines, which are safe and efficacious.
4. To employ traditional medicine practitioners in health services by means of skill-based and participatory approach training.

In an effort to extend the scope of health care services to rural and urban areas, traditional medicine was introduced in hospitals and clinics in all states and regions of Myanmar. There are now two 50-bed traditional medicine hospitals, twelve 16-bed hospitals and 237 district and township clinics. In addition, many private practitioners are also taking part in health care provision.

Traditional medicine in Myanmar is an inherited profession, interrelated with natural and climatic conditions, thoughts and convictions, and the social system. It is a broad, deep and delicate branch of science, covering basic medical knowledge, different treatises, a diverse array of therapies and potent medicine. Before 1976, the knowledge of traditional medicine was handed down from one generation to another. In 1976, with the aim of discouraging unqualified practitioners, the Institute of Myanmar Traditional Medicine was established and a systematic training programme was started to produce competent doctors. This three-year course conferred a diploma on the students, whose annual intake was about 100.

In 2001, the University of Traditional Medicine was established, which used modern learning methodologies in accordance with the systematic curricula, developed by the joint efforts of traditional practitioners and medical educationists. The curriculum covers the four *nayas*, basic science and concepts of Western medicine. This five-year course and one-year internship confers a Bachelor of Myanmar Traditional Medicine (BMTM) degree. The yearly intake is 175 students.

Since 2003, the basic concepts of traditional medicine were introduced in the curriculum of third year MBBS students. A module, comprising thirty-six hours of teaching and learning sessions of traditional medicine, was developed and incorporated together with assessment for completion. A certificate is given to all successful candidates. The main aim of the course is to familiarize medical students with this system of medicine. This type of teaching system, combining traditional and Western medicine, is the first of its kind anywhere in the world and paves the way for interested MBBS students to venture deeper into Myanmar traditional medicine.

Herbal Heaven

Myanmar's traditional medicine formulations are mainly based on medicinal plants. The country has been blessed with many species of herbs and vast tracts of vacant land where herbs can grow well.

With the main aim of perpetuating rare species of medicinal plants and producing raw materials for its factories, the Department of Traditional Medicine has been establishing one herbal garden after another. Since herbal gardening is still in its infancy, only 30 per cent of the area has been utilized at present. Herbal gardens are situated in different weather and soil conditions, so different species can be cultivated.

One of the biggest herbal gardens is the National Herbal Park which is 196.40 acres and located in the centre of Nay Pyi Taw. Its main aim is to enable people to observe available resources of Myanmar traditional plants in one place and preserve the endangered species.

According to Hundley and Chit Ko Ko, 1987, Myanmar has 1,524 species of medicinal and useful plants and 908 species of medicinal plants. The National Herbal Park has already collected 500 species of medicinal plants and 384 species are being cultivated there. The Park has now been establishing nurseries for medicinal plants which are used to treat diabetes, hypertension, tuberculosis, malaria, diarrhoea and dysentery.

The concerned ministries (i.e. Ministry of Health, Ministry of Progress of Border Areas and National Races and Development Affairs, Ministry of Agriculture and Irrigation, Ministry of Forestry) are collaborating with each other for the fulfilment of these traditional medicine objectives.

Traditional medicine is so important to Myanmar that the government is giving impetus to its development by systematically ramping it up to the international level and manufacturing potent medicines scientifically. Both public and private sectors are involved in manufacturing it, with two factories being run by the Department of Traditional Medicine.

The yearly production of each factory is 10,000 kg. and medicines are produced according to a national formula. In addition, these factories also manufacture twenty-one varieties in powder form which are given free to patients of public traditional medicine facilities. They also produce twelve kinds of drugs in tablet form for commercial purposes.

Due to the government's encouragement and assistance, the manufacturing of these medicines through correct methods and international level production processes, storage systems and packaging has enhanced public trust in the indigenous drugs and led to an increased demand.

The Research and Development Route

Myanmar has vast natural resources and biodiversity for strengthening scientific research. At the Department of Traditional Medicine, two typical Research and Development tasks are being carried out. The first is scientific analysis that involves implementation of research projects such as botanical, chemical, pharmaceutical, pharmacological and clinical investigations on traditional herbal drugs. Besides this, routine analysis on traditional drug samples for registration purposes, post-market drug survey and quality control for drug factories is being carried out.

Scientific research and analysis is being done to distribute safe and effective traditional medicines among people. At the same time, the monographs of Myanmar medicinal plants are being compiled and published in order to disseminate this knowledge throughout the world.

The second task is giving health education and training the people to rely on traditional medicines. For this, the Department publishes and distributes books, newsletters, magazines, posters and pamphlets. Efforts are being made to conserve old palm-leaf manuscripts which are written in Pali or Sanskrit and translated into Burmese.

A Law For Everything

To keep abreast of changing circumstances, the Department of Traditional Medicine reviewed and updated Myanmar Indigenous Medicine Act, 1953 and transformed it into Myanmar Traditional Medicine Council Law, which was enacted in 2000. One of the objectives of the Law was 'to supervise traditional medicine practitioners so that they abide by the rule of conduct and discipline'. At present, there are about 6,000 such registered practitioners. Licenses for practising are issued to those having a diploma in Myanmar traditional medicine or Bachelor of Myanmar Traditional Medicine.

In 1996, the government promulgated the Traditional Medicine Drug Law to control the production and sale of these medicines systematically. This was followed by a series of notifications concerning registration and licensing, labelling and advertising. One of the objectives of the Law was 'to enable the public to consume genuine, safe and efficacious quality traditional drugs'.

Under this Law, all traditional medicine drugs produced in the country have to be registered and the manufacturers must have licenses. There are now altogether 10,824 registered drugs and 2,150 licensed manufacturers.

Thanks to a market-oriented economic system and development of the economy, businessmen, tourists and scientists have visited Myanmar and taken an interest in its traditional medicine and natural resources. Samples of raw materials have probably been taken away to identify the ingredients in modern laboratories which will greatly benefit this system. Since there is no proper law to protect the intellectual heritage of Myanmar's traditional medicine and its property, there is an urgent need to do so. For this, meetings have been held on Intellectual Property Rights by various practitioners and manufacturers.

Protect this System

At present, we have the Traditional Medicine Drug Law and Traditional Medicine Council Law to protect this system of medicine. The former controls traditional drugs produced in the country so that its manufacturing is safe and efficacious. The Council Law enforces the professional and ethical practice of traditional medicine. Such a system will, it is hoped, protect Myanmar's traditional medicines.

Meanwhile, the Myanmar Traditional Medicine Practitioner Association was formed in 2002 to promote the potency and effectiveness of this system. The objective of the association is implementing programmes through the work of practitioners well-versed in their field, holding seminars in which the physicians seek means to revive hidden and extinct subjects, therapies and drugs and uniting all the practitioners of various groups under one banner. Another effort to propagate this system was started in 2000 with the Myanmar Traditional Medicine Practitioners Conference. Every year, practitioners from all over the country assemble here, exchange knowledge and hold discussions for the perpetuation and spread of this system.

In conclusion, Myanmar has striven for a modern and developed nation with healthy citizens who live in a green environment.

13

Mental Health Revisited

SUDHIR K. KHANDELWAL

MENTAL DISORDERS EXACT a profound economic and personal toll worldwide, yet public and private health care systems, particularly in developing countries, have paid little attention to them. Disabilities, along with premature deaths, caused by mental disorders comprise nearly 15 per cent of the burden of disease in developing countries.

A Chimera

For a long time, it was believed that serious mental disorders did not exist in India as we were a developing country, had our joint family system intact, and most of our population was religious and spiritual. All this was supposed to exert a protective influence on mental health. The proportion of people suffering from severe mental disorders was considered miniscule. Moreover, it was not considered worthwhile to invest the already scarce financial and manpower resources in looking after them.

However, since late 1970s, Indian epidemiological studies, as well as the WHO multi-centre collaborative study on severe mental illness, in 1974, have clearly demonstrated that the incidence and prevalence of mental disorders in India is no less than that in developed countries.

Globally, one out of four people suffers from a diagnosable mental illness in any given year. Approximately 3–5 per cent of the population may also suffer from a severe mental illness that can cause considerable dysfunction in their personal, familial, social and occupational functioning (World Health Report, 2001). This may also contribute significantly in pushing the family into poverty.

Mental disorders cause significant burden not only to the family, but also to the society as a whole. 'Global Burden of Diseases', a landmark study by Harvard University in association with the World Bank and WHO, clearly demonstrated that mental disorders contribute to considerable burden on a given nation, which is not any less than what is caused by other well-known diseases. The report showed that the total burden because of mental illnesses was approximately 11.50 per cent in 2004, and is likely to increase to 15 per cent by 2020. Moreover, it was seen that this is second only to what is caused by cardiovascular diseases, and more than that of cancer and HIV/AIDS. Thus, it means that mental disorders are more common and burdensome than tuberculosis, cancer, diabetes, HIV/AIDS, and blindness. The 2010 'Global Burden of Disease' study has reported that burden of mental illness and drug use has increased by 37.60 per cent between 1990 and 2010, which is a significant increase.[1] (Whiteford 2013).

Morbidity caused by mental illness can manifest itself in the form of disability, suicide, absenteeism, decreased productivity and higher labour turnover, accidents at work, family burden and most importantly, stigma. Behavioural problems caused by it can also have undesirable consequences like unsafe sex, increased alcohol, tobacco and drug use, road traffic accidents, violence and lifestyle disorders.

The grim message given by the epidemiological and the Harvard study was that the problem is huge, but we in India, or for that matter all developing countries, are not equipped to deal with it due to our meagre resources. Thus, the huge gap between needs and resources continues to impede us.

Health or mental health facilities, which are taken for granted in the West, are simply not available to large sections in India. The number of psychiatrists available within the country is approximately 4 per million as against 100 in the West. Similarly, it is 0.50 for psychiatric nurses (300 in the West), 0.30 for psychologists (140 in the West) and 0.30 for psychiatric social workers (150 in the West). Thus, India's yawning gap in terms of resources to deal with the increasing mental health burden is as much as 75 per cent.[2]

Thus, if India has to improve its mental health situation, it has to employ innovative ideas and solutions. It has a rich tradition of multiple systems that can contribute significantly to improving mental health and preventing the onset of these problems.

The Ancient Texts

India is a country that has a large number of traditional medicine systems, which are used and practised by many. Ayurvedic, Homoeopathic and Unani systems find easy acceptance here. Interestingly, India also has a tradition where non-pharmacological systems have always been advised for better health, particularly mental health.

A number of mental health professionals, like R. Srinivasa Murthy, N.N. Wig, A. Venkoba Rao, J.P. Balodhi, V.K Varma, and C. Shamsundar, have done studies and written extensively on the concepts taught in Indian philosophy, like the concept of mind, willpower and meditation. However, only a brief account is given of ancient Indian teachings on preventive and promotional aspects of mental health.

According to our ancient texts, a mentally healthy or ideal person is expected to govern his life in the utmost righteous way despite adversities. Shamsundar describes the mentally healthy person as the one who 'attends to one's legitimate duties in personal, family, social and occupational areas, fulfilling spiritual, affectional and material needs of self and family in harmony among one's role functions, one's abilities and limitations, prevailing circumstances and righteous means with sincerity and honesty, hope and confidence and contentment.'[3]

In the Vedas, the earliest scriptures written more than 5,000 years ago, we find that the mind is thought of as a functional element of *atman* and is treated as the sixth organ that controls the other five sense organs. It also controls and coordinates the impressions from the outside world, and enables thoughts and activities. In the *Rig Veda* and the *Yajur Veda*, *mantras* (rhymes) have been mentioned as a mode of prayer for enriching the mind with noble thoughts. In the *Rig Veda* (Chapter 1, Hymns 46, 48, 71, 76, 94), the speed of the mind, curiosity for methods of mental happiness, prayers for mental happiness and methods of increasing *medha* (intelligence) have been described. In the *Yajur Veda* (Chapter 34), the mind has been conceptualized as the inner flame of knowledge and has also been described as an instrument of knowledge and the basis of consciousness. In the *Atharva Veda*, the mind has been described as an instrument for hypnotism and in the sixth chapter, there is a detailed description of preservation of willpower, emotions, inspiration and consciousness. These same concepts continue in the Upanishads, which describe different states of mind such as waking, dreaming, deep sleep and *samadhi*. The *Bhagavad Gita* also presents a detailed account of human emotions and cognitive deviations, where the human mind and its weaknesses are elaborated. For example, the first mention of anxiety are in Ch. 1, Verses 29, 30, 31, when Arjuna, standing in the battlefield, describes his state as, 'my limbs are frozen, my mouth is dry, my body trembles and my hair stands on the end. Gandiva, the great bow, is slipping from my hand and my skin is burning. Nor can I stand up as my mind is whirling'.[4] From Chapter 18 onward, there is an emphasis on the methods to gain mastery over the vacillating mind and the consequences of failure to attain such mastery are also illustrated. Significant importance is given to attainment of self-knowledge, the Yoga of action or *karma*, knowledge of renunciation, importance of meditation, Yoga of devotion and wisdom of renunciation. The modern concept of cognitive restructuring has its base in the teachings of the *Bhagavad Gita*.

Traditional Systems

Ayurveda, said to be the science of life, has flourished in India and neighbouring countries for nearly 3,000 years. It is described as the science of positive health that teaches practices, rules and principles to ensure smooth running of intricate mechanisms of human mind and body. It deals with instructions regarding diet, work, rest and sleep; advocates a sense of purity, observation of sex hygiene and proper behaviour in general. It delineates methods for strengthening the body, and for its spiritual and mental development. The aim of Ayurveda is to help an individual to develop in harmony with his/her seasonal, climatic, social, religious and regional environment. It further advocates that to promote health and prevent diseases, there should be balance and harmony of the individual with the five elements (*panchbutta*), namely, water, fire, earth, air and sky; and the three humours (*tri dosha*), namely, *kapha* (phlegm), *pitta* (bile) and *vayu/vata* (wind). To achieve this, the person has to make conscious efforts to regulate his/her thoughts, speech and actions.

Yoga is another system for the mind. It evolved in ancient India several thousand years back as a means to attain *moksha*, or to unite with the supreme consciousness. Yoga can be deemed as a disciplined method utilized for attaining a goal, which is *moksha*. However, the exact definition of what forms *moksha* takes, depends on the philosophical or theological system with which it is conjugated. Bhakti schools of Vaishnavism combine Yoga with devotion to enjoy an eternal presence of Vishnu. In Shaiva theology, Yoga is used to unite *kundalini* with Shiva. The *Mahabharata* defines the purpose of Yoga as the experience of *brahman* or *atman* which pervades all things.

In the specific sense of Patanjali's *Yoga Sutras*, the purpose of Yoga is defined as *chitta-vitti-nirodha* (the cessation of the perturbations of consciousness). In contemporary times, the physical postures of Yoga are used to alleviate health problems, reduce stress and make the spine supple. Yoga is also used as a complete exercise programme and physical therapy routine. Patanjali Yoga that is practised to control the mind, is known as Raj Yoga. Yoga is the inhibition (*nirodha*) of alterations or modification (*vritti*) of mind (*chitta*). Patanjali's writing became the basis for a system referred to as Ashtanga Yoga or Eight-Limbed Yoga. The eight limbs are described as follows:

1. *Yama* (The five abstentions): *Ahimsa* (non-violence), *Satya* (truth), *Asteya* (non-covetousness), *Brahmacharya* (non-sensuality, celibacy) and *Aparigraha* (non-possessiveness).
2. *Niyama* (The five observances): *Shaucha* (purity), *Santosha* (contentment), *Tapas* (austerity), *Svadhyaya* (study of the *Vedic* scriptures to know about God and the soul) and *Ishvara-Pranidhana* (surrender to God).
3. *Asana*: Literally means 'seat', and in Patanjali's *Yoga Sutras*, it refers to the seated position for meditation.
4. *Pranayama* (Suspending breath): *Praana*, breath, *aayaama*, to restrain or stop. Also interpreted as control of the life force.
5. *Pratyahara* (Abstraction): Withdrawal of the sense organs from external objects.
6. *Dharana* (Concentration): Fixing attention on a single object.
7. *Dhyana* (Meditation): Intense contemplation of the nature of the object of meditation.
8. *Samadhi* (Liberation): Merging consciousness with the object of meditation.

In recent times, many scientific studies have been done to examine the efficacy of Yoga in health and disease. Various studies have shown that Yoga is beneficial for promoting mental health as well as in treatment of various physical and psychological ailments. For example, a recent study assessed the efficacy of Yoga by including seventy-seven subjects who either had ailments such as hypertension, coronary heart disease, diabetes, mild depression or were otherwise healthy but wanted to do Yoga for prevention of disease. It was seen that within two weeks, there was a significant difference in their state of subjective well-being, both emotionally and physically.[5]

Meditation

There are two fundamental attentional strategies. In Concentration Meditation, sustained attention is directed towards a single object or point of focus, without distraction, in order to produce a peaceful state of one-mindedness. We also have Mindfulness Meditation, where there is full awareness or mindfulness of any contents of consciousness with equanimity. Mindfulness meditation has now entered the health care domain and we have evidence suggesting a positive correlation between its practice and emotional and physical health. In one study seventy-six participants, diagnosed with anxiety disorders, were randomly exposed to either Mindfulness based therapy or the usual treatment. Significant improvement was seen in the former group of participants.[6] Systematic reviews of various studies that have assessed the effect of Mindfulness on various mental disorders such as depression, anxiety, addictions and even physical illnesses like heart conditions, diabetes, etc., strongly suggest the beneficial effect of Mindfulness in alleviating physical and psychological symptoms.[7]

Meditation has traditionally remained a practice for achieving the higher level of consciousness in man's quest for finding the supreme truth. It is usually practised along with Yoga. Meditation has been linked to a variety of health benefits. It may produce physiological benefits by changing neuro-cognitive processes. It has also been linked with various favourable outcomes that include: effective functioning (including academic performance), increase in concentration, perceptual sensitivity, decrease in reaction time, enhancement in memory, self-control, empathy and self-esteem.

To conclude, mental health is an important part of the agenda of health for everyone. In fact, there is 'No health without mental health' and 'If brain does not work, nothing else matters'. There is a huge burden on society due to mental health morbidity. To tackle it, it is imperative that measures be taken to prevent morbidity and promote mental health.

Our traditional systems, philosophy and spiritual practices have laid out definitive principles for promotion of mental health. By systematically following these practices at the individual or community level, it is reasonable to hope that there will be positive gains for mental health, reduction in morbidity and the consequent health burden.

Notes

1. H.A. Whiteford et al., 'Global Burden of Disease Attributable to Mental and Substance Use Disorders: Findings from the Global Burden of Disease Study 2010', *Lancet*, vol. 382, no. 9904, 2013, pp. 1575–86.
2. *Mental Health Atlas,* Department of Mental Health and Substance Abuse, World Health Organization, Geneva, 2011, <http://www.who.int/mental_health/evidence/atlas/profiles/ind_mh_profile.pdf>, accessed 16 January 2016.

3. Shamsundar, 'Relevance of Ancient Indian Wisdom to Modern Mental Health—A Few Sxamples', *Indian Journal of Psychiatry*, vol. 50, no. 2, 2008, pp. 138–43.
4. Shiv Gautam, 'Mental Health in Ancient India and Its Relevance to Modern Psychiatry', *Indian Journal of Psychiatry*, vol. 41, no. 1, 1999, pp. 5–18.
5. A. Sharma, *Spirituality and Mental Health*, Delhi: Indian Psychiatric Society in association with Rajayoga Education and Research Foundation, Mount Abu, 2008.
6. J. Vollestad et al., 'Mindfulness Based Stress Reduction for Patients with Anxiety Disorders: Evaluation in a Randomized Controlled Trial', *Behavior Research and Therapy*, vol. 49, 2011, pp. 281–8.
7. W.R. Marchand, 'Mindfulness Medication Practices as Adjunctive Treatment for Psychiatric Disorders', *Psychiatric Clinics of Northern America*, vol. 36, 2013, pp. 141–52; S. Netaji et al., 'Effect of Group Mindfulness-Based Stress-Reduction Program and Conscious Yoga on Lifestyle, Coping Strategies, and Systolic and Diastolic Blood Pressures in Patients with Hypertension', *Journal of Tehran Heart Centre*, vol. 10, no. 3, 2015, pp. 140–8.

References

Balodhi, J.P., 'Constituting the Outlines of a Philosophy of Ayurveda—Mainly on Mental Health Import', *Indian Journal of Psychiatry*, vol. 29, 1987, pp. 127–30.

Gautam, Shiv, 'Mental Health in Ancient India and Its Relevance to Modern Psychiatry', *Indian Journal of Psychiatry*, vol. 41, no. 1, 1999, pp. 5–18.

International Pilot Study of Schizophrenia, World Health Organization, Geneva, 1974.

Khandelwal, S. and K.S. Deb, 'Transcendental Meditation: Current Status', in *Psychotherapy in a Traditional Society: Context, Concept and Practice*, ed. V.K. Varma and N. Gupta, New Delhi: Jaypee, 2008, pp. 190–205.

Marchand, W.R., 'Mindulness Medication Practices as Adjunctive Treatment for Psychiatric Disorders', *Psychiatric Clinics of Northern America*, vol. 36, 2013, pp. 141–52.

Mental Health Atlas, Department of Mental Health and Substance Abuse, World Health Organization, Geneva, 2011, <http://www.who.int/mental_health/evidence/atlas/profiles/ind_mh_profile.pdf>, accessed 16 January 2016.

Netaji, S. et al., 'Effect of Group Mindfulness-Based Stress-Reduction Program and Conscious Yoga on Lifestyle, Coping Strategies, and Systolic and Diastolic Blood Pressures in Patients with Hypertension', *Journal of Tehran Heart Centre*, vol. 10, no. 3, 2015, pp. 140–8.

Rao, A.V., 'Psychiatric Thought in Ancient India', *Indian Journal of Psychiatry*, vol. 20, 1978, pp. 107–19.

———, *Culture, Philosophy, Mental Health*, Mumbai: Bharatiya Vidya Bhavan, 1997.

Reddy, S., 'Psychoanalytical Process in a Sacred Hindu Text: The *Bhagavad Gita*', in *Freud Along the Ganges: Psychoanalytical Reflections on the People and Culture of India*, ed. S. Akthar, New Delhi: Rave Media, 2008, pp. 308–34.

Shamsundar, 'Relevance of Ancient Indian Wisdom to Modern Mental Health—A Few Examples', *Indian Journal of Psychiatry*, vol. 50, no. 2, 2008, pp. 138–43.

Sharma, A., *Spirituality and Mental Health*, Delhi: Indian Psychiatric Society in association with Rajayoga Education and Research Foundation, Mount Abu, 2008.

Sharma, R., N. Gupta and R.L. Bijlani, 'Effects of Yoga Based Lifestyle Intervention on Subjective Well-Being', *Indian Journal of Physiological Pharmacology*, vol. 52, no. 2, 2008, pp. 123–31.

Srinivasmurthy, R., *Religion and Psychiatry: Beyond Boundaries*, ed. P.J. Verhagen et al., John Wiley & Sons Ltd., 2010, pp. 159–79.

The World Health Report, Mental Health: New Understanding, New Hope, World Health Organization, Geneva, 2001, <http://www.who.int/whr/2001/en/whr01_en.pdf>, accessed 14 January 2016.

Vahia, N.S., D.R. Doongaji and D.V. Jeste, 'Value of Patanjali's Concepts in the Treatment of Psychoneurosis', in *New Dimensions of Psychiatry: A World View*, ed. S. Arieti and G. Chrzanowski, New York: John Wiley & Sons Ltd., 1975, pp. 293–304.

Varma, L.P., 'Psychiatry in Ayurveda', *Indian Journal of Psychiatry,* vol. 7, 1965, pp. 292–312.

Vollestad, J. et al., 'Mindfulness based Stress Reduction for Patients with Anxiety Disorders: Evaluation in a Randomized Controlled Trial', *Behavior Research and Therapy*, vol. 49, 2011, pp. 281–8.

Weiss, M.G. et al., 'Humoral Concepts of Mental Illness in India', *Social Science & Medicine,* vol. 27, 1988, pp. 471–7.

Whiteford, H.A. et al., 'Global Burden of Disease Attributable to Mental and Substance Use Disorders: Findings from the Global Burden of Disease Study 2010', *Lancet*, vol. 382, no. 9904, 2013, pp. 1575–86.

Wig, N.N., 'Indian Concepts of Mental Health and Their Impact on Care of the Mentally Ill', *International Journal of Mental Health,* vol. 18, no. 3, 1990, pp. 71–80.

———, 'Mental Health and Spiritual Values: A View from the East', *International Review of Psychiatry,* vol. 11, 1999, pp. 92–6.

———, 'The Third-World Perspective on Psychiatric Diagnosis and Classification', in *Sources and Traditions of Classification in Psychiatry*, ed. N. Sartorius et al., Hogrefe and Huber Publishers, pp. 181–210.

———, *The Joy of Mental Health: Some Popular Writings of Dr N.N. Wig*, Chandigarh: Servants of the People Society, 2006.

14

Understanding
Mind-Body Relationships

VIJAYLAKSHMI
RAVINDRANATH

A S SCIENTISTS WE ARE often accused of working in isolation. It is said that we look at organs, cells, and molecular pathways in a segregated manner. This has been one of the major criticisms of modern biology and medical research and it is true to a certain extent. We have indeed often failed to look at the body as a whole, or even at the organs as a whole.

At the research front, we are now forced to think differently because we understand the complex interactions in the body—how the immune system, gut, GI and brain have a close interaction with each other and how one regulates and determines the outcome of the other. Even different systems of medicine could come to the same prognosis of an ailment.

Different Systems

Way back in 1996 at NIMHANS, Bangalore, there was an Indo-US meeting of Western psychiatrists and pharmacologists with Ayurvedic pundits such as Dr P.K. Warrier, Dr C.P. Joshi and Dr Dhondo Sadashiv Antarkar. The goal was to get both groups to talk about mental illness, starting from aetiology, diagnosis and treatment. After each physician had presented his view, two sets of physicians interviewed a patient with schizophrenia. This was recorded on video and shown to an audience.

The subject was interviewed separately by the psychiatrist and the Ayurvedic physician. It led to an important question—do both these systems of medicine with their different approaches lead to the same diagnosis of mental illness?

The Western psychiatrist enquired about the psychotic features while the subject was hallucinating rapidly. The Ayurvedic physician, however, asked him about his father. His father had an untimely death. This approach is the holistic one that we require today. Interestingly, an Ayurvedic physician from the audience watching the video said that the man must be diabetic just by looking at him and listening to him being interviewed by the Ayurvedic physician. And sure enough, he was.

So, there is no doubt that medicine should be holistic. Take for example, gut bacteria. What we eat influences what we are. The number of bacteria that colonize our intestine and body is actually greater than the number of cells we have. The number of genes that these bacteria produce are several fold more than the genes we have in our body. What we eat (probiotics, etc.) through this bacteria mediates and influences what we call the gut and the brain axis. So, the microbes in the gut actually influence the brain and behaviour through the endocrine system, through the vagus nerve and the immune system.

In fact, the gut micro-flora in depressive patients actually changes and that change is reflected in behaviour. If you take the micro-flora in autistic children, it is very different from what you see in normal kids. Incidentally, if you take rats and grow them in a germ-free environment where you do not have gut bacteria, it influences their behaviour. Similarly, probiotics reverse the influence of gut bacteria. Therefore, what we eat, which has been the fundamental tenet in our traditional systems of medicine, greatly influences cognition and behaviour.

So, if you have a healthy central nervous system, a healthy gut function, you will have normal behaviour, normal emotions and normal levels of inflammatory parameters. In diseased states, however, when there is an intestinal dysbiosis, it leads to alterations in behaviour and emotion. It also affects inflammatory parameters through the immune system.

Immune System

During stress, an axis starts from the brain—the hypothalamus, the pituitary, to the adrenal gland (HPA axis)—and regulates the secretion of an important molecule called corticosterone. This is a major mediator of the immune function, impacting behaviour during stress.

After acute stress, the brain sprouts more connections or spines, in certain instances. In experiments on rats, during acute stress, males actually perform better, whereas females lose spines.[1] But this just goes to show how a stress phenomenon actually produces a physical change in the brain in very short time periods, a few hours, in fact.

But during chronic stress, the paradigm changes, and both genders show marked differences. Males demonstrate a huge damaged area, whereas females survive it very well. This is probably because females have an adaptive response, considering they deal with chronic stress through pregnancy, childbirth and child-rearing.

Over the years, we thought the brain was isolated from the immune system. If you inject a foreign protein or a foreign bacteria into the body, you will see a huge immune reaction. But if you put that into the brain without too much of trauma, you do not see such an immune reaction. So, it was presumed that the brain was a closed box completely isolated from the immune system.

But more recently, it has been found that immune molecules are important in the development of synapse, which forms the connections in the brain. As new cells are produced in the brain throughout our lifetime, called neuro-genesis, it is actually the immune molecules that also regulate it. So the brain is no longer a box that is completely isolated, but is constantly in a vibrant interaction with the immune system, with both regulating each other.

If you have a depressed immune system and there is a high amount of inflammatory response, it has an impact on the brain. If you have stress, it will lower immunity. This constant interaction happens even during normal functions when the immune system builds and breaks connections. The brain is like a plastic organ, constantly changing, making new connections and breaking away. So, for neuroscientists, it is a challenge to look at the brain and see how it mediates behaviour and cognition. One has to holistically look at the gut, the immune system and the brain.

Alzheimer's Disease

Traditional knowledge can be used for new treatment strategies for Alzheimer's. Alzheimer's is a disease of ageing. According to Western data, nearly 40 per cent of people in their eighties develop Alzheimer's disease.[2] The disease was first described by Alois Alzheimer a century back when he met a fifty-one year old patient who was extremely psychotic. Later, she had a decline in memory. This loss of memory, disorientation and psychotic behaviour can have a devastating effect on the family. World Health Organization predicts that the incidence of Alzheimer's is going to be four to five folds higher in developing countries as compared to developed countries because of the sheer number of people who are over sixty years.[3] With increasing lifespan, this is going to be a huge public health problem.

India is not adequately prepared to deal with this issue as nuclear families do not have good support systems to take care of aged people. We do not have any drugs to treat Alzheimer's today. They are given only symptomatic treatment. That means we do not treat the disease, we do not cure the disease, and we do not even slow down the progression of the disease. It is like giving aspirin or saridon to a patient with a headache without understanding the cause of the headache and treating it.

It is a moot point if we can utilize the existing knowledge base for discovery and development of rational therapies for brain disorders. Dr V.P.K. Nambiar, an ethnopharmacologist, listed ten plants, which are used in *Medhya Rasayanas* in Ayurveda. Extracts were prepared from these plants by Professor S.C. Jain of University of Delhi and tested on transgenic mice with Alzheimer's disease mutations, so as to test their effect on the disease model (as per unpublished results from Dr Ravindranath's laboratory).

A small subsect of Alzheimer's patients carry a mutation which is passed on in a Mendelian inheritance manner, leading to a high preponderance of the illness in the family. These mutations are expressed in mice and they develop behavioural problems and the pathology seen in Alzheimer's disease. They are unable to negotiate a maze and have plaques in the brain. These animals were given these extracts and also a *gritham*, a ghee-based preparation. As one extract after another was given, it was noticed that the one from Aswagandha had a dramatic effect.

The experiment done on these mice was as follows. There were eight arms—four arms contained food. No more than four arms had the bait. The mice were trained to go directly into the arms that were baited and take the food. But the ones with the mutation did not know where to go. They wandered around and went to the wrong arm which did not have any food. But a month after giving the semi-purified extract orally, they finished the job without a single error.

These mice became calmer too. Normally, they were anxious. Further, when their brains, which earlier had plaques like Alzheimer's patients, were seen, the plaques had disappeared very dramatically. But surprisingly, it was found that the extract did not have an action on the brain. It instead acted on the liver, where it increased a protein called LRP which drew out the A-beta, a toxic molecule that causes most of the problems in Alzheimer's from the brain. This A-beta then is present in the blood and degraded by the liver and kidney.

There has never been a report so far that Alzheimer's can be treated by targeting the periphery, the liver, as we saw when we gave this plant extract. Dr Warrier said, 'Treat the body and the disease will be taken mind-body interaction will keep us healthy and help us age gracefully. It is time to talk more to traditional physicians and address childhood disorders as well. Traditional systems of medicines can contribute enormously in improving the health of children and aging adults and the devastating brain disorders they suffer from.

Notes

1. T.J. Shors, C. Chua and J. Falduto, 'Sex Differences and Opposite Effects of Stress on Dendritic Spine Density in the Male Versus Female Hippocampus', *J. Neurosci*, vol. 21, 2001, pp. 6292–7.
2. *2015 Alzheimer's Disease Facts and Figures*, Alzheimer's Association, accessed from <https://www.alz.org/facts/downloads/facts_figures_2015.pdf>.
3. *Dementia: A Public Health Priority*, World Health Organization, 2013.

15

Mind-Body Relationship in Diseases and its Management

RAMESH P.R.

ACCORDING TO AYURVEDA, health is the harmonious existence of physical, psychological and spiritual entities. This is equivalent to the World Health Oragnization's definition of health: 'It is complete physical, mental and social well-being.' The inseparable link between mind and body is always emphasized in Ayurveda for both preventive health care and treatment. Thus, its approach in addressing health issues is always psychosomatic in nature. According to Ayurveda, the functions of the brain can be summarized as follows:

- Place of soul (*Aatma*)
- Centre for consciousness (*Chetana*)
- Seat of special senses (*Pancha Jnanendriya*)
- Storehouse of intellect (*Buddhi, Medha*)
- Seat of subconscious mind (*Chitta*)
- Storehouse of memory (*Smriti*)
- Centre of life (*Jeevita*)
- Regulator of sleep (*Nidra*)
- Seat of emotion, passion (*Rajas*)
- Centre of 'Ego' Self-consciousness (*Ahankar*)[1]

Stress is an important factor that affects human life, positively and negatively. Stress is the body's response to any demand upon it. It is the general wear and tear of daily living.

Stressor: These are the demands and events that cause stress.

Eustress: This is good stress which is beneficial to life and helps in achieving goals.

Distress: This is excessive stress, destructive to physical, mental and emotional health.

All stress is not bad. It becomes a problem only when it becomes excessive and when we are unable to cope up with it. Our performance is directly connected with stress. The reasons for stress are many: daily hassles, changes in our environment, work, finances, relationships, conflict between people (interpersonal) and internal conflicts (intrapersonal). Each stressor is also addictive—a whole bunch of little stressors can add up to a large stress load. The concept of 'total pain' in cancer patients is an ideal example of the cumulative effect of stress as can be seen in Fig. 15.1

Reasons for Stress

Attachment of the mind to materialistic pleasures:

- Not getting desired things or experiences.
- *Icha*—Excessive desires.
- Not following a code of conduct.[2]

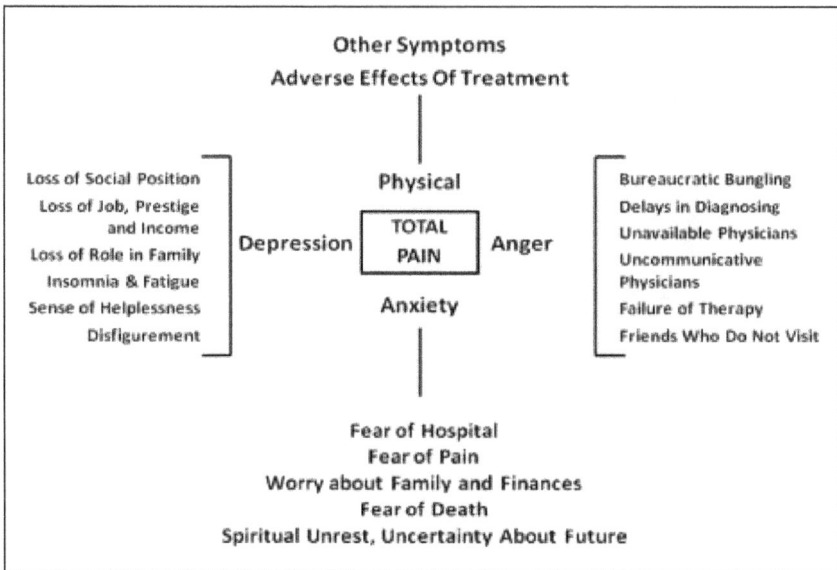

Fig. 15.1: The Concept of Total Pain.
Source: Robert Twycross, *Introducing Palliative Care*, Calicut, India: Institute of Palliative Medicine, Pain and Palliative Care Society, 5th economy repr., p. 66 (reproduced with permission).

Every action is aimed at one's well being. Well being cannot be achieved without deeds done with good intentions. So, one should strive to perform every action with good intentions only. This is the ultimate secret for better stress management.

Sukhartha Sarva bhutanam Matah sarvah Pravritayah
Sukham ca na vina dharmat tasmat dharma paro bhavet[3]

—*Ashtanga Hridayam, Sutram 2/20*

Understanding Stress

Stress is additive. The body's response to stress is the sum of all the stressful situations it is exposed to. Do not avoid stress. Keep it within manageable limits to use it to your advantage when possible. Also, note that stress is not 'out there', it is 'in here' within the person.[4] For the consequences of stress, see Fig. 15.2.

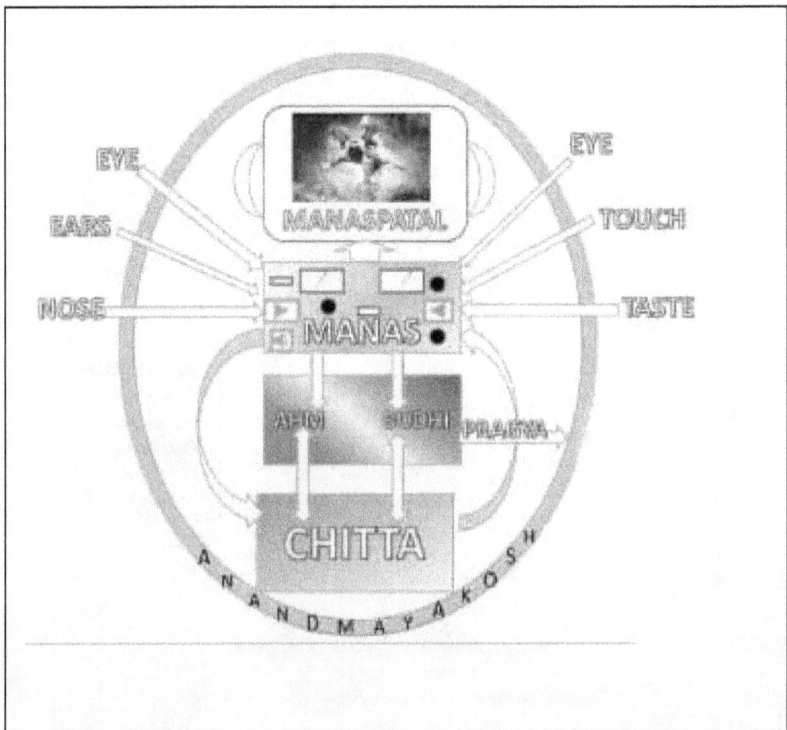

Fig. 15.2: Stress and Physiological Arousal.

Source: Study Materials, Hospital Management, Human Resource Management, Block-2, August 2009, National Institute of Health and Family Welfare, New Delhi, pp. 43–63; see especially p. 48 (reproduced with permission).

Symptoms of Stress

- Muscle Cramps   Stammering
- Skin turning white   Dryness/Paleness
- Lips turning blue   Butterflies in the stomach
- Fist gripping   Sweating
- Shakes/tremors   Nail biting
- Dilation of pupils   Loose motions
- Stimulated heart rate   Palpitations
- Fast breath   Body aches

Ailments caused by Stress

- Digestive and stomach disorders
- Sex problems
- Angina pectoris
- Peptic ulcer
- Ulcerative colitis
- Indigestion
- Constipation
- Respiratory psychogenic cough
- Bronchial asthmas
- Psychological impotence/Frigidity
- Obesity
- Diabetes
- Rheumatoid arthritis
- Headaches/Migraine
- Skin disorders
- Anxiety neurosis, Depression
- Psychogenic vomiting
- Rundown feelings or emotional problems
- Inexplicable fears[5]

Psycho-Neuro Immunology (PNI)

PNI[6] comprises of psychology, behavioural science, neuroscience, immunology, endocrinology, infectious disease, rheumatology, molecular biology, pharmacology, and also, physiological and psychiatric considerations. The physiology of hypothalamic-pituitary-adrenal axis, sympathetic adrenal axis and neuro-endocrines are important in physiological considerations. The effect of the response of the immune system is an important factor to be evaluated under PNI. For example, poorer antibody response in psychotic disorders, increase in pro-inflammatory cytokines in mood disorders, neuro-immune activation in neuro-psychiatric disorders and reduced NK cell lysis in sleep and stress related disorders are some of the responses that ought to be studied. Interpersonal relationships help to improve the positive response of immune system in cancer patients. For example, high quality emotional support from the spouse results in better NK cell activity in breast cancer patients.[7]

Stress generally induces immune suppression and a specific immune system response. Stress reduces apoptosis, alteration in DNA repair and NK cell activity. It is also responsible for lowering the levels of luteinizing hormone and testosterone concentrations. In a nutshell, stress can turn out to be either a 'killer' or a 'driving force' in terms of performance.[8]

Beating Stress

Adopt a healthy lifestyle. Bad habits such as smoking, skipping meals, late hours, etc., can increase stress.[9] So, get adequate rest, be physically active, eat regular, healthy meals, avoid smoking, alcohol, drugs, and relax, spend quality time with family and friends.

- *Do not over-commit*: Limit your demands, prioritize, and delegate.
- *Simplify life*: Inculcate habits to improve peace of mind.
- *Master one big change at a time*: Try to avoid too many changes in one go. When going through major life events, try to keep other changes that are within your control to a minimum. Major life events include new job, marriage, divorce, new home, death of a loved one, serious illness, etc.
- *Learn to relax*: Relaxation is the antidote for stress.
- *Be physically active*: This burns up pent-up emotions, relaxes the muscles, improves sleep, distracts you from problems, improves mood and thereby improves resistance to stress.
- *Be good to yourself*: Listen to self-talk, build your self-esteem, make changes where needed.
- *Feed your emotional life*: Everyone needs love to survive and cope with life. Do not isolate yourself.
- Resolve conflicts by improving communication skills, respecting other's views. Improve assertion skills by being direct and honest.

Keep balance in life by improving the quality of spiritual intelligence. The eight signs of spiritual intelligence are:

1. Flexibility
2. Self-awareness

3. Ability to face and use sufferings
4. Tendency to probe and ask fundamental questions
5. Ability to be inspired by a vision
6. Ability to work against convention
7. Ability to see connection between diverse things and thinking holistically
8. A desire and capability to cause as little harm as possible[10]

Laughter and music therapy, Yoga, meditation, prayer and Ayurvedic treatments based on *Panchakarma* are effective in the management of stress.[11] There are nine commandments given by Acharya Vagbhata for good health. These are as follows:

Nityam hitaraviharasevee sameekshyakaree vishayeshvashkata/
daata, sama, satyapara
kashamavam aptopasevi ca bhavatyarogh

—*Ashtanga Hridayam, Sutram* 4/36

It means: 'One who enjoys wholesome food and activity everyday; who introspects on his action; who is unattached; who is generous; who looks on all with an equal eye; who is truthful and forgiving; who delights in the service of virtuous men; He remains free from illness.'[12]

Notes

1. *Charaka Samhita, Sutrastana*, vol. I, Chapter 8, Slokas 1–35; Dr Ram Karan Sharma and Vaidya Bhagwan Dash, Chowkhamba Sanskrit Studies, pp. 163–82.
2. Ibid.
3. *Sukhartha Sarva Bhutanam Matah Sarvah Pravritayah,* collated by Dr Anna Moreswar Kunte and Krishna Ramachandra Sastri Navre, Krishnadas Academy, 1995, p. 29.
4. 'Stress', *Home Health Information Medical Reference Guide*, University of Mary Land Medical Centre, USA, pp. 1–23.
5. Ibid.
6. Ibid.
7. Janice K. Kiecolt-Glaser et al., 'Stress, Personal Relationships, and Immune Function, Health Implications', *Brain, Behaviour and Immunity,* vol. 13, 1999, pp. 61–72.
8. Perikedem et al., 'Department of Psychology and Department of Science', *Psychology and Health,* vol. 6, no. 3, July 1992, pp. 159–73.
9. *Home Health Information Medical Reference Guide,* pp. 1–23.

10. Study materials, Hospital Management, Human Resource Management, Block-2, August 2009, National Institute of Health and Family Welfare, New Delhi, p. 53.

11. M.S. Valiyathan, *Susruta Samhita, Sutram* 1/27, *The Legacy of Susruta,* Orient Longman, 2007.

12. M.S. Valiyathan, *Ashtanga Hridayam, Sutram* 4/36, *The Legacy of Vagbhata,* University Press, 2011.

16

Mind-Body Relation in Ayurveda

C.R. AGNIVES

I N AYURVEDA, THE living being, be it man, animal or plant, is an integral whole. Division of this whole into parts such as the body and the mind is only for academic purpose, as none of these components can operate separately.

Living It Up

The term *purusha* can be easily misunderstood as it has different connotations in different contexts, sciences and even common languages. In Ayurveda, *purusha* means a living thing. However, in the context of human medicine, it means a living human being. In the case of equine medicine (*asvaayurveda*), it means the horse and in the case of plant medicine (*vrkshaayurveda*), it refers to the plant. In short, *purusha* can mean any living thing.

A person is divided into two parts: sentient and non-sentient. The former, also called *chetana*, is non-material, substantial and existent. In common parlance, we may term it 'life'. Thus, the person has life and body. The non-sentient part has five existents (five elements). The body is non-sentient (*achetana* or *jada*) and inert as any other non-living thing. It is only in combination with the sentient that the body can function as a living being.

Both the sentient and the body can be further subdivided. The two parts of the sentient are soul (*atman*) and mind (*manas*). The sentient nature of the mind is a reflection of the sentient nature of the soul. Soul is sensory and motor. It is the knower and doer. The mind is only a tool in the hands of the soul for collecting knowledge and doing things. The mind is active like a screwdriver or spanner in the hands of the mechanic. It is the mechanic who decides the action of the tool. Being a mere tool, the mind does not have any will. Desire, aversion, etc., are the properties of the soul and not of the mind. The division of the sentient into mind and soul is absent in contemporary Western psychology, where the psyche is seen as a solitary, indivisible entity.

As mentioned earlier, the inert body is made up of five existents (*panchabhuta*). The body can also be divided into two—the body proper and the faculties. The faculties are sensory receptors and motor instruments. They are known as *indriya* in Sanskrit. They are also made up of five existents. Though the body is inert, the faculties exhibit more sentient nature during life than the body proper, as they function only in conjunction with the mind which is conjugated with the sentient soul. It is like light passing from an illuminated room through a door to someone sitting outside. Thus, in Ayurveda, the living thing is a continuum with four components—soul, mind, faculties and the body proper.

The mind is a super faculty (*atindriya*) as it is a combination of the sensory and the motor. There are five sensory and five motor faculties. There are eleven faculties in total, including the mind. But the mind is an internal faculty (*antarindriya*) which can communicate with the exterior only through other faculties which are external. They are called *baahyindriya* as they come in contact with external things which are their objects.

In Ayurveda, sense organs such as eyes and nose are not considered faculties. They only form the abode of the various faculties. Faculties are minute and imperceptible. They can only be inferred from their function, just like the mind.

There are five sensory faculties and hence, there are five pentads to be known (*indriya-pancha-panchakam*). Each pentad consists of five things:

- Faculty
- Object
- Sense organ
- Substance having the object
- The sense or knowledge generated through the faculty

The five pentads are given in Table 17.1.

TABLE 17.1: The Five Pentads

Pentads	Faculty (existent)	Object	Sense Organ	Substance	Sense or Knowledge
1	Auditory	Sound	Ear	Ether	
2	Tactile	Touch	Skin	Air	
3	Visual	Colour	Eye	Fire	
4	Gustatory	Taste	Tongue	Water	
5	Olfactory	Smell	Nose	Earth	

The 11 faculties and their functions are listed below:

• Sensory faculties

1. Auditory faculty   To receive sound
2. Tactile faculty   To receive touch
3. Visual faculty   To receive vision
4. Gustatory faculty   To receive taste
5. Olfactory faculty   To receive smell

• Motor faculties (represented symbolically)

1. Grasping faculty (hand)   To grasp and hold
2. Locomotor faculty (foot)   To move about
3. Excretory faculty (anus)   To expel wastes
4. Communicative faculty (tongue)   To communicate
5. Reproductive faculty (genitals)   To reproduce

• Sensory-motor faculty

1. *Mind*: To think, to receive information and to direct actions

The Mind

The mind is conceptualized as the thinking faculty in Ayurveda. Its job is to contemplate, collect information, and present facts to the soul, akin to a private secretary. Once a decision or action is taken by the boss, the private secretary sees it through by engaging sense faculties to collect objects. These are ideas which are thought of or contemplated. These are presented to the soul, which then decides what to do or not to do. Accordingly, the mind engages the motor faculties to get things done.

But should there be a mind? Is it possible for the sentient to collect information directly? It is not because like the mechanic or carpenter, the soul cannot act without tools. The mind and faculties are its tools. Without them, the soul is unable to perceive knowledge and thus unable to act.

Can the soul directly contact the faculties? This is not so because it will only create confusion as more than one faculty will get connected with the soul and lead to superimposition of information at the cost of clarity. Imagine many films being projected on the same screen at the same time. It will be very confusing. To avoid this, there should be a controller to select the faculty, one at a time. There should be strict discipline here. The mind has to see that only one faculty gets connected with the soul at any given time.

While the mind is not the knower, it is the main tool for collection of knowledge. To perceive, the sense object should get connected with the sensory faculty, the sensory faculty with the mind and the mind with the soul. In life, mind is always in union with the soul. When we are absent-minded, this flow is impossible. Hence, in Ayurveda, the mind is defined as the cause of knowledge and ignorance. When the mind is linked in the sequence of information chain, there is knowledge and when unlinked as in deep sleep, there is no information. In a wakeful state, the mind is always linked with some faculty. It may also engage in itself for contemplation and appear absent-minded.

In Ayurveda, the mind is considered to be minute. Similarly, there is only one mind in a person. If there are many minds, superimposition of information will occur. Some consider the heart (*hrdaya*) as the seat of the mind, others consider it to be in the brain (*siras*). In fact, in Sanskrit, *hrdaya* is used as a synonym for the mind. *Bhela-samhita*, a classical text of Ayurveda, mentions that the heart is situated between the vertex and the palate. This indicates the brain. Heart is also considered to be the seat of the sentient.

Omnipresent Mind

The mind is everywhere in the human body. It is in each living cell as each cell has to take its decisions. But as a multicellular organism, the mind of man should have a central control. There should be a collective mind for this purpose. That is why we think of a collective mind and its seat.

In Ayurveda, there is a heart-brain axis, representing the functions of the mind. Though the actual process of thinking is taking place in the brain, the effect of thinking is expressed by the heart. Increase and decrease of heart rate due to mood changes are evident in the muscular heart. This fact caused the notion that the mind functions in the heart.

Being a silent organ without palpable movement, nothing much is mentioned about the brain in Ayurveda. This does not mean that Ayurveda is unaware of the brain. The head is the superior most organ as it is the seat of *praana*, the most important faction of the humor *vata*, which controls all nervous operations and the mind.

The main object of the mind is to think. This may be subdivided into many processes. Anything that can be thought of is the direct object of the mind. Thinking includes thought (*chintyam*), contemplation (*vicharyam*), deduction (*oohyam*), meditation (*dhyeyam*), imagination (*samkalpyam*), etc.

According to Indian philosophy, the whole universe has three major attributes—*sattva* (knowledge), *rajas* (action) and *tamas* (ignorance). This is from the psychological viewpoint. We can have only three emotions—love, hatred and confusion. Love is knowledge or one that causes knowledge, even though in common parlance, we consider love to be blind. Hatred or aversion causes action meant to avoid the object of aversion. When we do not know whether to love or hate, we are confused. To be or to not be is the state of confusion.

In other words, man has desire (*ichaa*). Desire to have something is love. Desire not to have something is aversion (*dvesha*). But when we cannot decide whether to have or not or whether to act or not, there is confusion (*moha*). Since all things are capable of creating love, hatred and confusion, we conclude that there are elements of love, hatred and confusion in each and everything in the universe.

Why the Confusion?

Take the case of a rose. When you know the flower, you are happy and love it. But if the flower reminds you of some unhappy instance or person or causes some kind of allergy, you would wish to avoid it. But if you do not know what the flower means, then you are confused. So, the flower has all the factors of love, hatred and confusion.

Confusion causes fear and inertia. Hatred causes agony and pain. Love causes affection. Let us examine a case. A small child is presented with a moving, colourful toy which makes sound. At first, the kid may be afraid of the toy and may even cry if it is thrust on him. He is averse to it and will push it away. Later, when he knows the toy, he will desire it and be happy with it.

The mind is capable of developing fear, anger and confusion because it also possesses the three attributes and is part and parcel of the universe. At any given moment, the predominance of *sattva, rajas* or *tamas* dictates whether you are happy, unhappy or confused. The major attributes (*tri guna* or *maha guna*) are interconvertible. Hence, *sattva* can change into *rajas* or *tamas* and vice versa. Their major attributes are as follows:

- *Sattva* causes a sense of hygiene, theism and fondness for good and benevolent deeds.
- *Rajas* causes talkativeness, pride, anger, aversion and competition.
- *Tamas* causes fear, ignorance, inertia, sleep, laziness and a depressive mood.

While *sattva* is considered pure, the other two are considered to be pollutants of the mind. They are malevolent, colour the information passed through the mind and mislead the soul. In mental diseases, both *rajas* and *tamas* work together to generate symptoms.

According to Ayurveda, many diseases, usually considered mental diseases, such as psychosis, have a physical bearing and are classified according to the humours, viz., *vata, pitta* and *kaph*. The cause of mental diseases is considered as guilt complex generated by an intellectual error termed as *prajnaa-aparaadha*. An intellectual error is an act which is inconsiderate of proper judgement *(dhee)*, self-control *(dhrti)* and memory *(smrti)*, culminating in an inauspicious end. However, if such an act culminates in auspiciousness, it is not considered as an aetiologic factor.

Another concept is that mental diseases are caused by the unavailability of the desired and presence of the undesired, i.e. the loss of things one is fond of and the presence of hated things. Treatment of mental diseases consists of generating correct knowledge, improving self-control and generating orientation. Orientation includes time orientation, place orientation and personal orientation.

Mind-Body in Tandem

Only a healthy body can lodge a healthy mind. Hence, Ayurvedic treatment of mental diseases includes purification of physical humours and their subsequent mitigation by internal medicine and physical medicine.

At any given moment, there will be a predominance of any one of the three attributes in the mind. The person will then be considered as belonging to that mental temperament. Thus, mental temperaments are classified into three—*sattvika, rajasa* and *tamasa.* These may be translated as pure, arrogant and ignorant mental temperaments. There are many subdivisions to these and they are named after mythological characters, animals and plants. But these are just examples and there can be innumerable subdivisions. Physical constitution is permanent in a person. But mental temperament may change due to experiences and intentional efforts.

Psychosomatic and somato-psychic relation is well understood in Ayurveda. It is stated that the ailments of the mind will pass on to the body and vice versa. For example, in fever, which usually is a physical disease, we find mental symptoms such as laziness, somnolence, lack of attention, inversion of preferences, and aversion to sound, etc., even in the prodromal stage. Hemiplegia may cause behavioural errors. Mental diseases like madness may also have organic basis. Many physical diseases have psychic factors as a sound aetiology. In classifying physical diseases, Ayurveda has given a slot for psychological types. Thus, we have descriptions of fever due to fear, anger, worry, lust, etc. There is diarrhoea due to fear and grief and vomiting due to dislike.

The relation between the mind and the body is illustrated by the example of a metal vessel and ghee. Hot ghee poured into a cold vessel will heat up the vessel. On the other hand, cold ghee poured into a heated vessel also will get heated up. Such is the relation between mental and physical diseases.

There is no consideration of the mind without the body in Ayurveda. Phenomena like clairvoyance are manifestations of an abnormal mind and have no reality as per Ayurvedic philosophy. Even though transmigration of soul is considered in Ayurveda, it is appended with the mind and a minute body (*sukshma-sharir*). Hence, in life and even in life after death, mind is in constant relation with the body until it achieves absolute liberation called *moksha.* The mind is, therefore, part and parcel of the living body and in life, it is constantly influencing it.

References

Ashṭaangga-hṛdaya of Vaagbhaṭa II with Sarvaanga Sundara, commentary by Arunadatta.
Ashṭaangga-saṃgraha of Vaagbhaṭa I with Ṣaṣilekha, commentary by Indu.
Bhela-samhita by Bhela.
Charaka Saṃhita by Agnivesa with Ayurveda Deepika, commentary by Cakrapaani.
Maadhava Nidaana of Maadhavakara with Madhukosa.
Pandita, Ṣreedaasa, *Hṛdaya-bodhika Commentary of Ashṭaangga-hṛdaya.*

Saarngadhara-samhita, commentary by Aadhamalla.
Susruta-samhita by *Suśruta* with *Nibandhasaṃgraha,* commentary by Ḍalhana.

List of Publications by Late Professor C.R. Agnives

Adhunika Dampatya Sastram (Marriage Manual) in Malayalam.
Ayurvedeeya Rasasastram (Book on Mineral Treatment) in Malayalam.
Ayurvedic Medical Procedures in English (forthcoming).
Darsana Pravesika (Book on Philosophy of Ayurveda) in Malayalam.
Dravyaguna Vijnanam (Ayurvedic Pharmacology), 2 vols., a co-authored work published by the Government of Kerala, from English to Malayalam.
Glossary of Ayurveda, a short glossary originally written in English and translated by Mariam L. Salganik in Russian, Moscow: NAAMI Medical Center.
Lessons on Ayurveda, a computerized interactive course for foreign students (to be launched by KAL) in English.
Rogavijnanavum Vikriti Vijnanavum (Principles of Ayurvedic Pathology), a co-authored work published by the Government of Kerala, from English to Malayalam.

17

Mind and Body

Interrelated and Interdependent

P.N. TANDON

I N ASIAN COUNTRIES, a great emphasis is laid on mind-body
interaction and harmony as an essential element for promoting human
health. For centuries, the various systems of health care in these
countries have included a variety of practices to achieve a holistic approach
for promoting health and preventing diseases (*Charaka Samhita* 79:54).[1]

Modern Medicine

Conventionally, modern medicine refers to the Allopathic system of
medicine. It is only during the last couple of decades that the practitioners
of Allopathy have come to recognize the role of lifestyle as a causative
factor, especially for heart disease, diabetes, metabolic syndrome and more
recently, in the aetiology of cancer. A recent report from USA claims that
our lifestyle is to be blamed for 70 to 90 per cent of cancer cases. Thus,
high calorie intake, especially fibre deficient carbohydrates, excessive fat,
lack of green vegetable and fruits, coupled with sedentary existence and
lack of exercise are responsible for ill health of a vast majority of people
in recent times.[2] To this may be added smoking and use of other forms
of tobacco, excessive intake of alcohol and other drugs of addiction. A
study from Oxford published recently in the *American Journal of Clinical
Nutrition* has reiterated that vegetarians have been found leading a healthier
life as compared to non-vegetarians. A balanced diet was considered a
prerequisite for healthy living in Ayurveda.[3]

The mind and body are interrelated and interdependent on each other. The two should function in harmony to ensure good health. We should look at our heritage, culture, religion, ethics, aesthetics and customs as true determiners of our lifestyles. This is the point which was greatly emphasized in our ancient system of medicine—the Ayurveda.[4] But we often forget this and adopt lifestyles which result in bodily discord and diseases. Under a variety of influences, we have changed some of our time-tested practices in favour of so-called 'modern' and 'civilized' ones, leading to adverse effects on our health. Mahler, then Director General of World Health Organization, in a lecture at the All India Institute of Medical Sciences on 10 January 1989, pointed out that 'health' was not even included as a subject in the medical curriculum. Fritjof Capra in his book *The Turning Point: Science, Society and Rising Culture* commented, 'Many people obstinately adhere to the biomedical model of disease because they are afraid to have their lifestyle examined and to be confronted with unhealthy behaviour' (as a cause of ill health).[5] Modern medicine, till a decade ago, completely forgot the relationship of lifestyle with health and disease. In contrast, as its name indicates, Ayurveda is the Science of Life—a holistic system of health promotion and care. The main aim of Ayurveda is to live a life which is free from physical and mental disorders.[6] Many of our customs are neither codified nor empirically tested. However, they have been passed on from generation to generation and have withstood the test of time. They should not be dismissed as primitive or obsolete under the influence of Western culture.

Ancient Knowledge

History is replete with examples of how societies have either been forced to or have voluntarily acquiesced their own time-tested customs in favour of unsubstantiated claims of other cultures. It was Jawaharlal Nehru who remarked that Ayurveda and Unani are repositories of great ancient knowledge, deserving our respect.[7] But all this has to be put to scientific tests. This is one of the reasons because of which we have lost much of our valuable heritage.

Let us take the case of Ayurvedic pharmaceutics. They are in the form of pills, decoctions, tinctures, creams, etc., which have their own specific use for different indications. Our country woke up only recently and realized that there should be a proper multidisciplinary effort to study this system. This involves the Council of Scientific and Industrial Research, the Indian Council of Medical Research, and AYUSH, which deals with Ayurveda, Unani, Siddha and Homoeopathy.

As for the Ayurvedic system, little is known of its active principle in decoctions. If you try to identify the active principle and then test it, the actions are different. For instance, Dr Bhusan Patwardhan, a scientist from Pune University, published a paper where he spoke about testing animals with the extract of *semecarpus anacardium*, a native plant of India, known as a cancer preventive agent. He found that it was quite useful. But when he used the active principle, it had no action at all.[8] Therein lies the constant struggle between practitioners of modern medicine and those of Ayurveda. In the Ayurvedic system, there are very precise methods which are to be followed to achieve the desired results—right from where you get the herb, how long it has to be stored and how it is to be produced as a drug.

I am more interested in another aspect of Ayurveda, which is the *Rasayantantra*. It deals not just with prevention or cure of a disease, but also with enhancing health. Many drugs are used in it, but more importantly, the whole system tells us what to eat, how much to eat, how much to rest, and how to spend our lives.[9]

Spiritual Therapy

Charaka, the father of Ayurveda, said that there are three types of therapy, namely, spiritual, rational and psychological. William James, supposed to be the father of modern psychology, said that faith can affect both physical health and disease process, and certainly, the mind.[10] However, it was only in 1984 that the WHO accepted the idea that the spiritual component is the fourth ingredient of mental health. Until recently, health professionals have sought to treat patients by focusing on medicine and surgery only. But now, physicians and patients have started realizing the value of faith, hope and compassion in the healing process. It is not surprising then that in most cultures in the ancient times, medicine was practised by clergies, saints and religious personnel.

Spiritual values are unique and different from religious values. Spirituality is often defined as a belief in the ultimate reality. It acknowledges the existence of a supreme power or spirit. It strives towards achieving the feeling of transcendence, strengthening the inner world and harmonizing interpersonal relationships.

An individual's physical and mental health is subservient to the spiritual self. Faith and spirituality have a profound and lasting effect on personality, immune system and mental health. An interesting study done among African-Americans who had a strong relationship with God, found that they were less likely to report depressive symptoms as compared to those who did not have such a bond.[11] Another study, done in 2002 by Larry Culliford, a consultant psychiatrist in UK, found that even though many see religion and medicine as peripheral to each other, spirituality and clinical care belong together. In another study, 93 per cent of cancer patients said that it was religion which sustained their hopes.[12]

The practice of Yoga, meditation and self-surrender to the Supreme Being have a definite role in psychotherapy, especially in behavioural medicine. Although Yoga was developed for spiritual upliftment, and not for therapy, during the last fifty years, it has been observed that Yogic practices help in maintaining health. Regular practice of Yoga is beneficial in the management of stress disorders.[13]

Benefits of Yoga

Clinical Yoga has been practiced in India since the dawn of human history. Millions of enthusiastic believers of this ancient tradition are found all over the world today. Modern scientific research has established its value for promoting all aspects of human health—physical, mental and spiritual.[14]

A number of renowned physicians have found modern medicine inadequate in several respects. They then looked at the ancient systems of medicine and utilized special Yogic practices for conditions as diverse as hypertension, myocardial infraction, depression, neurosis and chronic pain. Dr Selvamurthy, Director of Life Science in Defence Research and Development Organization (DRDO) and my erstwhile colleague Dr S.C. Manchanda, systematically studied the use of Yoga in patients who were angiographically diagnosed to be suffering from coronary artery disease.[15] They found that Yoga delayed the progression of disease, and even reversed the existing atherosclerotic lesions in coronary arteries. The effect of Yoga breathing exercises (*pranayam*) on airway reactivity in subjects with asthma has been observed.[16]

Diet and Health

There is also a link between food and health. Our ancient systems laid as much emphasis on food and lifestyle as on the use of drugs, meditation and exercise.[17] The food we took in our childhood was far superior to what we consume today. In my childhood, we used coarse grains in our daily diet. We gave up these coarse grains which had good fibre and adopted the polished rice and white flour. What did we get? Hypertension, diabetes, colitis and constipation. Similarly, in my childhood, it was understood that a newborn should be reared on mother's milk. Suddenly, powdered milk came in a tin. This was very convenient and was followed by many. We ought to realize what damage we do to our children, when we leave natural products.

I conclude with a statement by Einstein:

Let all of us therefore summon our strengths, let us be tirelessly on guard lest it be said later of the intelligent elite of this land: Timidly and without struggle they surrendered the heritage handed down to them by their forefathers, a heritage we were not worthy of. Let us rise, learn from each other and by coming together, we certainly can find many common grounds which can now be studied properly, scientifically and their value established.

Notes

1. Shiv Sharma, '*Charaka Samhita* 79:54', *The System of Ayurveda*, Bombay: Shri Venkateshwar Steam Press, 1929.
2. H.C. Trowell and D.P. Burkitt, *Western Diseases, their Emergence & Prevention*, London: Edward Arnold, 1981.
3. P.N. Tandon, 'Human Health and Our Heritage', in *In the Indian Human Heritage*, ed. D. Balasubramanian and N. Appaji Rao, Hyderabad: Universities Press (India) Ltd., 1998.
4. Shiv Sharma, *The System of Ayurveda*.
5. Capra.
6. G.P. Dubey et al., *Brain Ageing and Ayurveda*, New Delhi: Central Council for Research in Ayurveda and Siddha, 2008.
7. Jawaharlal Nehru, *Speeches Delivered at the Annual Sessions of the Indian Science Congress,* ed. Baldev Singh, New Delhi: Nehru Memorial Museum and Library, 1986.
8. B. Patwardhan, 'The Quest for Evidence-Based Ayurveda: Lessons Learnt', *Current Science*, vol. 102, 2012, pp. 1406–17.
9. Dubey et al., *Brain Ageing and Ayurveda*.
10. William James, *Textbook of Psychology*, London: Macmillan, 1903.
11. R.K. Wallace, 'Physiological Effects of Transcendental Meditation', *Science*, vol. 167, 1970, pp. 1751–3; L. Cacioppo, 'In Report of a Study by Scientist at the University of Chicago', *Times International*, 2005; C. Holden, 'Subjecting Belief to Scientific Methods', *Science*, vol. 284, 1999, pp. 1257–9; M. King, P. Speck and A. Thomas, 'The Royal Free Interview for Religious and Spiritual Beliefs', *Psychological Medicines*, vol. 25, 1995, pp. 1125–34; P.N. Tandon, 'Belief: A Scientific Perspective', in *Expanding Horizons of the Mind Science(s)*, New York: Nova Science Publishers, 2012, pp. 21–32.
12. Seamus Hayes, 'Spirituality and Clinical Care', *British Medical Journal*, vol. 325, 2002, pp. 1434–5.
13. H.K. Koenig, M.E. McCullough and D.B. Larsen, *Handbook of Religion and Health*, Oxford: Oxford University Press, 2001; P.N. Tandon, 'Belief: A Scientific Perspective', pp. 21–32; idem, 'Religion and Health', in *Science and*

Spirituality: The Growing Interface, New Delhi: Sri Sathya Sai International Centre for Human Values, 2012, pp. 155–60.

14.   J.C. Pearce, *The Biology of Transcendence*, Rochester, Park Street Press, 2002; R.J. Davidson, 'Alternation in Brain and Immune Functions Produced by Mindful Meditation', *Psychosomatic Medicine*, vol. 65, no. 564, 2003; S. Telles, 'Neural Plasticity and Yoga', in *Consciousness and Genetics*, ed. S. Menon, A. Sinha and B.V. Sreekantan, Bangalore: National Institute of Advanced Studies, 2002, pp. 275–82; R.K. Wallace, 'Physiological Effects of Transcendental Meditation', *Science*, vol. 167, 1970, pp. 1751–3; H. Herzog et al., 'Changed Pattern of Regional Glucose Metabolism During Yoga Meditative Relaxation', *Neuropsychobiology*, vol. 23, 1990, pp. 181–7; J. Khusu et al., 'Frontal Activation During Meditation Based on Functional Magnetic Resonance Imaging (FMRI)', *Indian Journal of Physiology and Pharmacology*, 2000, quoted by Telles; S. Telles, 'Neural Plasticity and Yoga', pp. 275–82; A. Newberg et al., 'The Measurement of Regional Cerebral Blood Flow During Complex Cognitive Task of Meditation: A Preliminary SPECT Study', *Psychiatry Research*, vol. 106, 2001, pp. 113–22; A. Lutz, Greischar, L.L., Rawlings, N.B. et al., 'Long-Term Mediators Self-Induce High Amplitude Gamma Synchrony During Mental Practice'; Y.W. Kuboto et al., 'Frontal Midline Theta Rhythm is Correlated with Cardiac Autonomic Activities During Performance of an Attention Demanding Meditation Procedure', *Cognitive Brain Research*, vol. 11, 2001, pp. 281–7.

15.   W. Selvamurthy et al., 'Physiological Responses of Cold (10 degree C) in Men After Six Months Practice of Yoga Exercise', *International Journal of Biometeorology*, vol. 32, 1988, pp. 188–93.

16.   V. Singh et al., 'Effect of Yoga Breathing Exercises (Pranayam) on Airway Reactivity in Subjects with Asthma', *Lancet*, vol. 335, 1990, pp. 1381–3.

17.   Tandon and Gopinath 1984; Tandon, 'Human Health and Our Heritage', pp. 22–4.

References

Bijlani, R.L., 'Dietary Fibre: Consensus and Controversy: Progress in Food and Nutrition', *Science*, vol. 9, 1985, pp. 343–93.

Bijlani, R.L. et al., 'Glycaemic and Metabolic Responses to a Traditional Cereal-Legume Mixture', *International Journal of Food Science and Nutrition*, vol. 44, 1993, pp. 243–51.

Burkitt, D.P. and H.C. Trowell, eds., *Refined Carbohydrates Foods and Disease: Some Implications of Dietary Fibre,* London: Academic Press, 1975.

Cacioppo, L., 'In Report of a Study by Scientist at the University of Chicago', *Times International*, 2005.

Davidson, R.J., 'Alternation in Brain and Immune Functions Produced by Mindful Meditation', *Psychosomatic Medicine,* vol. 65, no. 564, 2003.

Dubey, G.P. et al., *Brain Ageing and Ayurveda*, New Delhi: Central Council for Research in Ayurveda and Siddha, 2008.

Hayes, Seamus, 'Spirituality and Clinical Care', *British Medical Journal*, vol. 325, 2002, pp. 1434–5.

Herzog, H. et al., 'Changed Pattern of Regional Glucose Metabolism During Yoga Meditative Relaxation', *Neuropsychobiology*, vol. 23, 1990, pp. 181–7.

Holden, C., 'Subjecting Belief to Scientific Methods', *Science*, vol. 284, 1999, pp. 1257–9.

James, William, *Textbook of Psychology*, London: Macmillan, 1903.

King, M., P. Speck and A. Thomas, 'The Royal Free Interview for Religious and Spiritual Beliefs', *Psychological Medicines*, vol. 25, 1995, pp. 1125–34.

Khusu, J. et al., 'Frontal Activation During Meditation Based on Functional Magnetic Resonance Imaging (FMRI)', *Indian Journal of Physiology and Pharmacology*, 2000.

Koenig, H.K., M.E. McCullough and D.B. Larsen, *Handbook of Religion and Health*, Oxford: Oxford University Press, 2001.

Kuboto, Y.W. et al., 'Frontal midline theta rhythm is correlated with cardiac autonomic activities during performance of an attention demanding meditation procedure', *Cognitive Brain Research*, vol. 11, 2001, pp. 281–7.

Lutz, A., Greischar, L.L., Rawlings, N.B. et al., 'Long-Term Mediators Self-Induce High Amplitude Gamma Synchrony During Mental Practice', Proceedings of the National Academy of Sciences, USA, vol. 101, no. 46, 16369–73, 2004.

Manchanda, S.C., 'Retardation of Coronary Atherto-Sclerosis with Yogic Practice', *General Association Physician India*, vol. 48, 2000, pp. 687–94.

Nehru, Jawaharlal, *Speeches Delivered at the Annual Sessions of the Indian Science Congress*, ed. Baldev Singh, New Delhi: Nehru Memorial Museum and Library, 1986.

Newberg, A. et al., 'The Measurement of Regional Cerebral Blood Flow During Complex Cognitive Task of Meditation: A Preliminary SPECT Study', *Psychiatry Research*, vol. 106, 2001, pp. 113–22.

Patwardhan, B., 'The Quest for Evidence-Based Ayurveda: Lessons Learnt', *Current Science*, vol. 102, 2012, pp. 1406–17.

Pearce, J.C., *The Biology of Transcendence*, Rochester: Park Street Press, 2002.

Selvamurthy, W. et al., 'Physiological Responses of Cold (10 degree C) in Men After Six Months Practice of Yoga Exercise', *International Journal of Biometerology*, vol. 32, 1988, pp. 188–93.

Sharma, Shiv, *The System of Ayurveda*, Bombay: Shri Venkateshwar Steam Press, 1929.

Singh, V. et al., 'Effect of Yoga Breathing Exercises (*Pranayam*) on Airway Reactivity in Subjects with Asthma', *Lancet*, vol. 335, 1990, pp. 1381–3.

Tandon, P.N., 'Belief: A Scientific Perspective', in *Expanding Horizons of the Mind Science(s)*, New York: Nova Science Publishers Inc., 2012, pp. 21–32.

———, 'Religion and Health', in *Science and Spirituality: The Growing Interface*, New Delhi: Sri Sathya Sai International Centre for Human Values, 2012, pp. 155–60.

———, 'Human Health and Our Heritage', in *The Indian Human Heritage*, ed. D. Balasubramanian and N. Appaji Rao, Hyderabad: Universities Press (India) Ltd., 1998.

Telles, S., 'Neural Plasticity and Yoga', in *Consciousness and Genetics*, ed. S. Menon, A. Sinha and B.V. Sreekantan, Bangalore: National Institute of Advanced Studies, 2002, pp. 275–82.

Trowell H.C. and D.P. Burkitt, *Western Diseases, their Emergence & Prevention*, London: Edward Arnold, 1981.

Wallace, R.K., 'Physiological Effects of Transcendental Meditation', *Science,* vol. 167, 1970, pp. 1751–3.

Index

Aristotle 23
Arivu 34–5
Arivudambu 39
Arkan 25
Arteries 36, 156
Arthritis, rheumatoid 41
Arusuvai 42
Asana 107
Ashtanga Yoga 107
Ashta ragam 41
Asia xv, xvi, 88
    medicine systems in xvi
Asian medicines xv
Astangahrdaya 62
Asthma xv, 90, 156
Astral body 8
Astringent 42, 85
Atharam 39
Atharva Veda 105
Athithya mandilam 40
Aththi 36
Atindriya 146
Atman 3, 8, 105–6, 145, *see also* Soul
Atomic theory of Kanada 19
Augendiagnostik 72
Austerity 40–1, 107
Avalambakam 44
Avarice 41
Avaththai 39, 42
Awareness 9, 13–15, 55–6, 71, 108,
    120
    mental 55–6
    self- 15
Ayurveda xv–vi, 18–19, 24–6, 29–30,
    54, 59, 62, 106, 114, 116, 123–9,
    132–3
    dhatu systems 19
Ayu samuthan 50
AYUSH 90, 154
Aza 25
Azhal 36, 40, 43–4
    types of 43

Baahyindriya 124
Bachelor of Myanmar Traditional
    Medicine (BMTM) 99
Balodhi, J.P. 105
Barnard, Dr Christian 18

Behaviour 51, 55, 57, 59–60, 62, 81,
    106, 112–13, 132
    body 81
    ethical 62
    moral 59
    unhealthy 132
    verbal 59
    violent 51
Behavioural therapy 59, 62
Belly 49
Bhagavad Gita 105–6
Bhajan 12
Bhautik 23
Bhesajjamañjusá 59
Bhesijja 96
Bhog yoonis 2
Bible 3, 5, 15
Bile 23, 25, 50, 59–60, 65–6,
    106
Biology 20, 28–9, 31, 111, 119
Biomolecular Western medicine 28
Birth and death
    afraid of 4
    barrier of 5
    cycles of 41
    fear of 4
    forms of 47
    human 6, 12, 35, 47
    mysteries of 5
    phenomenon of 8
    physical process of 9
    previous 41
    successive 41
Bitterness 42
Black bile 23, 25, 59
Bladder 34, 38, 70
Blood 19, 23, 39, 42–3, 50, 59–60,
    65–6, 70, 80–2, 95, 114
    vessels 39, 81–2
Body
    aspects of xvi
    astral 8
    behaviour 81
    causal 11
    corporeal 25
    energy 8–9
    functioning of xv, 25, 44, 50
        physiological 44

Lungs 34, 38, 44–5, 70, 75, 83
Lust 41, 151
Lying 30, 41, 62

Macharyam 41
Madness 41, 58, 129
Madras Registration of Practitioners of
    Integrated Medical Act of 1956
    89
Mahabharata, the 106
Mahabhutas 24–6, 30
    corporeal 26
Maharaja Charan Singh 6
Malakkudal 38
Malam 39–40, 44
Malaria 85, 99
Malavasayam 38
Malaysia 33
Male 42, 45
Malevolence 57–8
Manam 35, 38–9
Manas 9–10, 26, 123
Manaspatal 9–10
Manavudambu 39
Mandilam 39–40
Manipulation 27, 52
Manipurakam 39
Mann 34, 42, 45
Manomayakosam 39
Manomaya Kosha 8, 30
Mantras 46, 105
Manu 6
Manuscripts 33, 100
    palm leaf 33
Marma 19
Marrow 19, 39, 42, 65
Mars 34
Maruts 6
Massage 51–2, 71, 76
    therapy 52, 71
Materialization 30
Matham 41
Maulana Rum 13
Maya 8, 12
Mayai 40
Medha 116
Medhya Rasayanas 114
Medical ethics 48
Medical knowledge 49, 98

Medical system xv–vi, 33, 49, 52, 54,
    64–5, 67, 84–5, 88, 92–3
    Buddhist and 54
    indigenous xvi, 54
    modern xvi, 33
    Tibetan 64, 67, 93
    traditional system
        Chinese xvi, 48
        forms of 93
        Indian xvi, 48
        Myanmar xvi
        Sri Lankan xvi
        Thai xvi, 49
        Tibetan xvi
Medicine
    Allopathic xv, 131
    Asian xv
    Chinese 50
    effective xvi, 97
    emergency 69
    Greek 26
    holistic 31
    Indian 23
    modern 18–19, 131, 133–4
    potent xvi
    prophetic 27
    psychiatric 26
    psychosomatic 26–7
    selection of 81
    Siddha system of 33
    spiritual dimension of 27
    system of xv, xvii, 19, 33, 48, 89, 91,
        93, 97, 99, 101, 111–12, 131–2,
        134
        ancient 33, 132
        traditional 97
        ancient xvii, 134
        Chinese 19
        Indian 33, 89
    traditional xv, 21–2, 26–31, 48–9,
        97–102, 105
        anatomy of 21
        Myanmar xv, 97, 99, 101
        optimization of 31
        Thai xv
        Tibetan xv
    Unani 22–7, 29–31
    Western 26, 28, 30–1, 49, 99
        biomolecular 28

www.ingramcontent.com/pod-product-compliance
Lightning Source LLC
Chambersburg PA
CBHW031537260326
41914CB00032B/1853/J

* 9 7 8 9 3 8 4 0 9 2 7 4 0 *